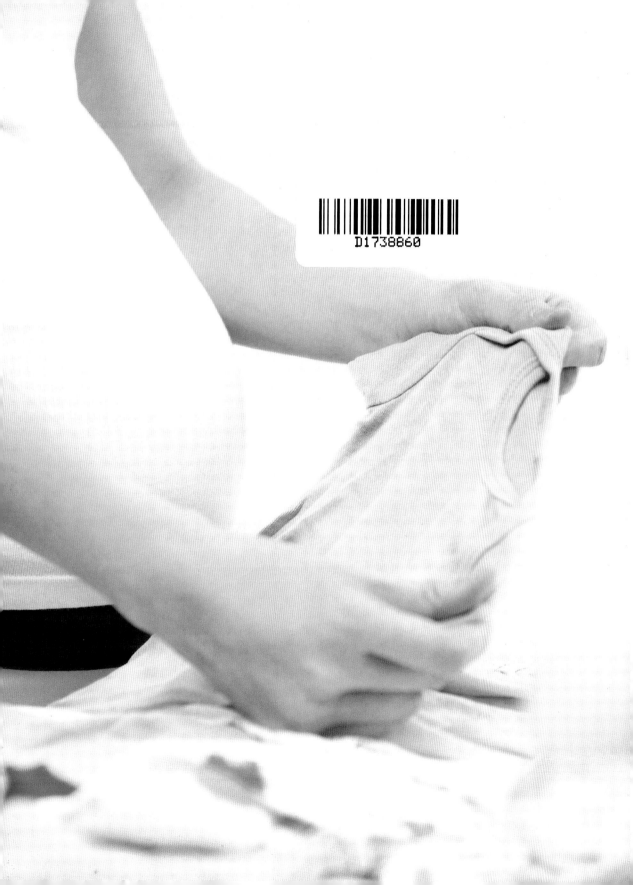

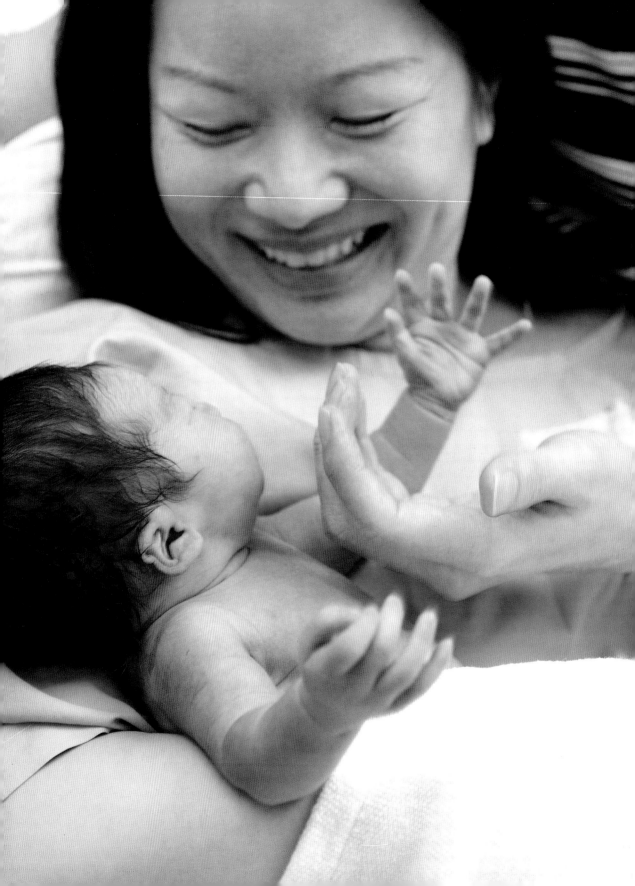

The Essential Guide for
First-time
Asian
Mums and Dads
from Pregnancy to Preschool

Dr Peter Chew, Mrs Kathleen Chia, Dr Chng Seo Yi, Dr Chong Shang Chee,
Asst Prof Linda Gan, Ms Anna Jacob, Sr Kang Phaik Gaik, Dr Jennifer Kiing,
Dr Yvonne Ng, Prof Quak Seng Hock, Dr Pamela Sharpe, Assoc Prof Lynette Shek,
Dr Wendy Sinnathamby, Dr Mas Suhaila Isa and Ms Gloria Chan

with a Foreword by Assoc Prof Daniel Goh

This book is supported by
an educational grant from

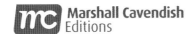

Marshall Cavendish
Editions

Abbott

A Promise for Life

Editor   : Lydia Leong
Designer   : Lynn Chin Nyuk Ling
Photographers : Joshua Tan, Elements By The Box and Liu Hongde (pages 94–95)

This book is supported by an educational grant from Abbott Nutrition.
All royalties from the sale of this book will be donated to the Singapore Children's Society.

Published by Marshall Cavendish Editions
An imprint of Marshall Cavendish International
1 New Industrial Road, Singapore 536196

Marshall Cavendish International (Asia) Private Limited,
1 New Industrial Road, Singapore 536196
Tel: (65) 6213 9300   Fax: (65) 6285 4871
E-mail: genref@sg.marshallcavendish.com
Online bookstore: http://www.marshallcavendish.com

The publisher makes no representation or warranties with respect to the contents
of this book, and specifically disclaims any implied warranties or merchantability
or fitness for any particular purpose, and shall in no events be liable for any loss of
profit or any other commercial damage, including but not limited to special, incidental,
consequential, or other damages.

Other Marshall Cavendish Offices:
Marshall Cavendish International. PO Box 65829 London EC1P 1NY, UK
• Marshall Cavendish Corporation. 99 White Plains Road, Tarrytown NY 10591-9001,
USA • Marshall Cavendish International (Thailand) Co Ltd. 253 Asoke, 12th Flr,
Sukhumvit 21 Road, Klongtoey Nua, Wattana, Bangkok 10110, Thailand • Marshall
Cavendish (Malaysia) Sdn Bhd, Times Subang, Lot 46, Subang Hi-Tech Industrial Park,
Batu Tiga, 40000 Shah Alam, Selangor Darul Ehsan, Malaysia

National Library Board, Singapore Cataloguing-in-Publication Data

The essential guide for first-time Asian mums and dads : from pregnancy to preschool /
Peter Chew ... [et al.] ; with a foreword by Daniel Goh. – Singapore :
Marshall Cavendish Editions, c2011.
p. cm.
Includes bibliographical references and index.
ISBN : 978-981-4276-68-9

1. Parenting – Asia. 2. Child rearing – Asia. 3. Pregnancy – Asia.
4. Child development – Asia. I. Chew, Peter, Dr.

HQ755.8
649.1095 -- dc22   OCN693758967

Printed and bound in Singapore by KWF Printing Pte Ltd

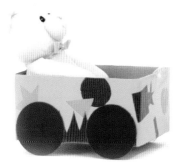

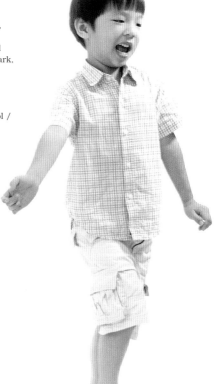

Acknowledgements

This book would not have been possible without the combined efforts of:

Assoc Prof Daniel Goh and his team at the Department of Paediatrics at the National University Hospital: Dr Chng Seo Yi, Dr Chong Shang Chee, Dr Jennifer Kiing, Dr Yvonne Ng, Prof Quak Seng Hock, Assoc Prof Lynette Shek and Dr Mas Suhaila Isa.

Dr Peter Chew, senior consultant obstetrician and gynaecologist at Gleneagles Medical Centre and Chairman of aLife, Sr Kang Phaik Gaik, senior lactation consultant at the Parentcraft Centre at Mount Alvernia Hospital, and Dr Wendy Sinnathamby at the Raffles Children's Centre at Raffles Hospital; Mrs Kathleen Chia, Asst Prof Linda Gan and Dr Pamela Sharpe, early childhood education specialists; and writer Gloria Chan.

The team at Marshall Cavendish International (Asia) Pte Ltd, Chris Newson, Violet Phoon, Sanae Inada, Lydia Leong, Lynn Chin; and photographers Joshua Tan and Liu Hongde.

The team at Abbott Nutrition International, Hui Hwa Koh-Minjoot and Anna Jacob.

Thanks are also due to the families, doctors, hospitals and mother and baby supply stores who assisted in this publication:

Alvernia Parentcraft Centre and Delivery Suite, Mount Alvernia Hospital • Delivery Suite, Gleneagles Hospital • University Children's Medical Institute, National University Hospital • Dr Chan Poh Chong, Senior Consultant, National University Hospital • Dr Ernest Lim, Anesthesiologist, Gleneagles Hospital • Baby's Hyperstore • Mums & Babes Pte Ltd • Alan, Fatima, Sharifah Nicole and Anna Sofia Chou • Paul, Su, Sophia and Scarlet Cantwell • Jeron, Lervanda and Dillon Chew • Chin Wei Chong, Ying Ying and Shuang Heng • Chow I-Ruh • Andy, Lydia and Ernest Goh • Gu Jing • Sanae Inada • Lee Swee Kay, Hwee Cheng and Kai En • David and Dorothy Leong • Jane Low • Desmond, Yumi, Kyrie and Kezia Ng • Ng Kok Wei, Mui Hoon and Megan • Nur Un Nissa • Reese, Linda, Jordan and Carter Seah • Mave, Jolynn, Maecia and Marcus Soh • Tan Ah Thai, Le Thi Kim Thuy, Tan Hui Ying and Tan Hui Juan • Khai Munn, Jolene and Jarius Sze Toh • John, Karen, Bella Rose and Lola Jane Wilkinson • Yap Guan Heng, Xu Jun and Dione

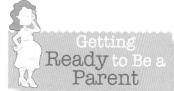
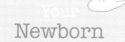
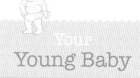
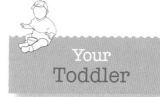
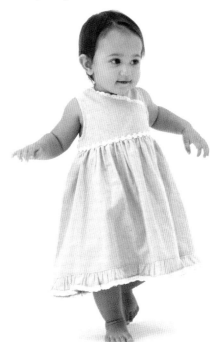

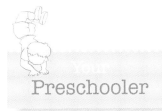

Your Preschooler

The Child with Special Needs

Health Care and Safety

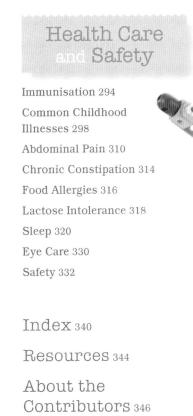

Foreword

Congratulations on picking up this book. The fact that you are reading this indicates that you are interested in learning more about raising children, and this is certainly an important first step towards successful parenthood.

Bringing up a child is challenging, yet fun and exciting. The different phases of childhood present different needs which need to be dealt with using different strategies. The learning process should start even before the baby is born. Preparation is important to give you a head start on the road to parenthood. Important aspects of infant and child care, such as cultivating good sleep habits and feeding routines, can have a significant impact on the subsequent life of your child.

Illnesses in early childhood can be stressful, especially for new parents. Being informed enables you to look out for signs and symptoms that may pose serious problems. Preventive health care through vaccination is vital and with the increasing numbers and varieties of vaccines available today, having a clear understanding and appreciation of the roles (and also adverse effects) of each vaccine is important for every parent.

Simple routines such as feeding and weaning to toilet training and disciplining the child can vary widely across cultures. Traditional and folklore beliefs also play a significant part in each family and can sometimes be a source of conflict between generations. Having reliable references based on good clinical and scientific evidence, which you will find in this book, would certainly be helpful in these situations.

The increasingly competitive education system has significantly increased the demands on the school-going child. Parents often add to the pressure with the good intention of 'helping' the child maximise his potential. What parents need to know are the ways to encourage, nurture and stimulate their child and to focus on identifying talent without overwhelming him. At the same time, parents should be sensitive to detect the subtle signs of learning and behavioural disorders and seek appropriate attention if need be.

Understanding and relating to your child through the growing years requires you to appreciate the social and emotional developmental milestones and to assist your child in developing his moral values and beliefs. Most important of all, you will have to provide a stable and loving home environment for your child.

The challenging process of raising a child never actually ends even though the relationship between you and your child will evolve through the years. But you will soon discover that parenthood is the most rewarding and fascinating experience of your life.

Assoc Prof Daniel Goh
Head of Paediatrics & Senior Consultant
University Children's Medical Institute
National University Hospital, Singapore

President
Singapore Paediatric Society

Vice-President
College of Paediatrics and Child Health, Singapore

Introduction

Are you thinking about having a baby or are you already expecting a baby? If your answer is "yes" to either question, you must be eagerly anticipating the day you will hold your precious little one in your arms. Yet, once in a while, you may also wonder if you will ever be up to the task. You are not alone.

Having a child will definitely change lives—yours, your spouse's and your family members'. It has been said that "a baby will make love stronger, days shorter, nights longer, bankroll smaller, home happier, clothes shabbier, the past forgotten and the future worth living for."

As a parent, you will want the best for your child. All your hopes and ambitions will be channelled to focus time and energy into nurturing and nourishing your child. This is one task you want to do well. And you know there is little room for failure as you will get only one chance to do it right. However, your baby will not come with a manual.

Some learn their parenting skills on the job, others by observing their own parents and still some pick up the ropes by reading avidly. There is no one sure shot way of doing it right. And what worked for one generation or family may not be right for this generation or your family.

There is so much to know and do. Parents need to cover all aspects of care, from ensuring optimal nutrition for their child's physical and mental development to providing opportunity, time, space and equipment for play and learning, and ensuring appropriate social, emotional and moral development for their child.

Parenting is a challenge—physically, mentally, emotionally and socially—but it is truly an enriching and joyful one. The smile on your baby's face when he sees you; his tiny hand gripping your finger as he sleeps; his coos, gurgles and babbles; the wiggle of his body as he tries to turn himself over, then as he learns to crawl and takes his first baby steps are all indelible milestones that will enrich your life as a parent. You are set to begin one of the most amazing experiences in life. The deep bond of love that will bind you to your child is one that will help you embrace the challenges and enjoy the thrills and spills throughout the journey of parenting.

To celebrate your plunge into the exciting life as a parent and to provide you with a tool to walk through the early days, months and years of parenting, Abbott Nutrition is glad to support this first local, comprehensive, up-to-date and complete guide written by more than a dozen top professionals in the fields of obstetrics, neonatology, paediatrics, nutrition and education.

Whether you choose to read it all at once to get an overview of what to expect or read it chapter by chapter as you traverse the different phases of parenting, the information within these pages will provide you with valuable nuggets of advice to give your child the very best in life.

All royalties from the sale of this book will go to the Singapore Children's Society. So, apart from getting the very best information available today from the experts in Singapore when you buy this book, you will also be helping an underprivileged child.

Hui Hwa Koh-Minjoot
General Manager
Abbott Nutrition International, Singapore

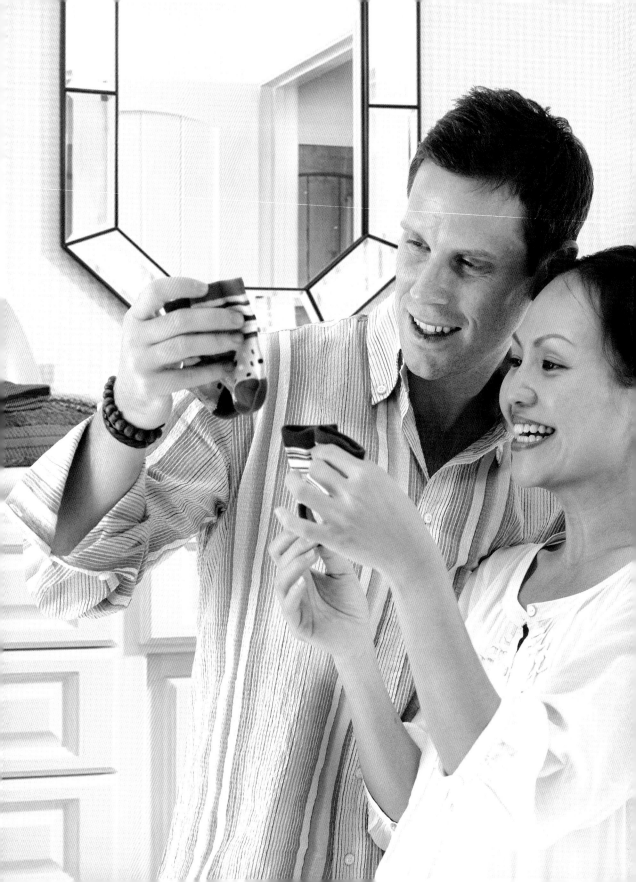

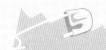

Getting Ready to Be a Parent

Becoming a parent is one of the most
exciting and challenging experiences in life.
And knowing what to expect as you and your spouse
start to plan a family goes a long way towards easing
your anxiety and preparing you for the time ahead.
So as you ready yourselves to become parents,
read up as much as you can and check with
your doctor if you have any doubts or queries.

Contributors:

Dr Peter Chew
Ms Anna Jacob

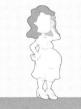

Pregnancy   0 to 1 month   2 to 11 months   12 months to 3 years   3 to 6 years

Preconception Care

If you are planning to have a baby, preconception care is important. This involves assessing the woman's overall health and identifying and being aware of any problems that might affect the mother and baby. Preconception care should ideally begin a year before conception. Make an appointment with your doctor for a preconception medical assessment.

Medical History

During your preconception medical assessment, you will be asked to give a detailed medical history of any chronic medical conditions. For example, if you suffer from high blood pressure or diabetes, you will be advised to get it under control before you conceive to reduce the risk of any problems in your pregnancy. In some cases, your medication may have to be adjusted or replaced with other treatment before you become pregnant. Because of your medical condition, you may need special care during pregnancy.

Past surgical history, especially surgery involving reproductive organs, hernia repair and appendectomy (removal of the appendix), is also important as this may affect your fertility.

You will also be asked in detail regarding past pregnancies, complications such as high blood pressure, gestational diabetes, premature labour, premature birth, birth defects and pregnancy losses (miscarriages and stillbirths). Share any concerns or fears you may have with your doctor. If you had a problem in a past pregnancy, it does not necessarily mean the problem will recur. Most women go on to have normal pregnancies and healthy babies.

Genetic Disorders

Inform your doctor of genetic disorders that run in your family. Based on your age, family history and ethnic group, genetic screening and counselling can help you find out your risk of having a child with a birth defect and give you the opportunity to discuss the options.

Immunisation for Preventive Care

If you are planning to have a baby, talk to your doctor about immunisation. Check that you have the following vaccinations as these will help protect you and your unborn baby against the following diseases.

- Measles, Mumps, Rubella (MMR) vaccine
- Varicella (chickenpox) vaccine
- Human papillomavirus (HPV) vaccine
- Hepatitis A vaccine
- Hepatitis B vaccine
- Pneumococcal vaccine

Vaccinations

Let your doctor know if you have had previous vaccinations, especially German measles, hepatitis B and chickenpox. Vaccinations can prevent some infections and it is important to be vaccinated before becoming pregnant as some vaccines are not safe for you during pregnancy.

Contraception

You will also be asked about the method of contraception you use. If you have been taking birth control pills, you will be advised to stop taking them two to three months before trying to conceive to allow your uterus to go through normal cycles before you become pregnant.

Sexually Transmitted Diseases

If you are at risk of sexually transmitted diseases (STDs), you should inform your doctor as these can increase the risk of infertility, ectopic pregnancy (when the fertilised egg implants outside the uterus) and other pregnancy complications.

If you think you or your spouse may have an STD, get tested and treated right away. Neither of you should have sex until treatment is complete. Infection with human immunodeficiency virus (HIV) can be harmful to the mother and baby. Early treatment may help prevent the infection from being passed on to the unborn baby. Because of this, your doctor will offer HIV testing even if you have no symptoms.

Lifestyle Habits

It is important to live a healthy lifestyle when you want to become pregnant. Discuss with your doctor your diet plan, exercise regime and how to manage your stress level.

Avoid alcohol, tobacco and illicit drugs as these substances can cause infertility. Your spouse's lifestyle too can also affect your pregnancy. Some studies have found that if your spouse smokes, drinks or uses drugs, it can lower his fertility by damaging his sperm. Living with someone who smokes also means that you are likely to breathe in harmful amounts of second-hand smoke.

Preparing for Pregnancy

Pregnancy, however well planned, still comes as a surprise. If you are waiting to change your lifestyle—to eat better, start exercising and stop smoking and drinking alcohol—after you know you are pregnant, it may be too late. There is evidence that shows that the quality of a woman's diet during pregnancy has an influence on foetal and maternal outcomes. Therefore, a healthy, balanced diet is important before as well as during pregnancy, and it makes good sense to prime your body for pregnancy.

Weigh in Right

A healthy body weight improves a woman's chances of conception. Being overweight or underweight makes it harder for a woman to conceive. Having an overweight spouse also lengthens time to conception.

Starting pregnancy at a healthy weight lowers the risk of complications for you and your baby such as hypertension, gestational diabetes, caesarean-section, preterm labour and delivery, and stillbirth.

Work with a dietitian or nutritionist to give your diet a makeover.

* If you are overweight, make careful food choices to reduce energy intake while ensuring that your diet delivers all the vital vitamins and minerals needed for optimal nourishment. Do regular exercise to burn calories. Keep going until you see the weighing scale moving towards your ideal weight for height.

* If you are underweight, you need to add portions of nutrient-rich food to step up the total energy content of your diet. If you cannot eat a lot more at mealtimes, then add nourishing snacks. Keep up your regular exercise but do not increase the time, intensity or duration. This will help you build up a caloric fund that should translate into weight gain over time.

Maternal Nutrition and Foetal Development

The developing foetus is most vulnerable to the mother's nutritional status during the first eight weeks, typically before pregnancy is confirmed.

New evidence also suggests that poor maternal nutrition may lead to changes (reprogramming) in the genetic materials within the foetal tissues and this predisposes the infant to chronic illnesses in adulthood.

Fill the Nutrient Gaps

Many adults know about healthy eating but a close look at their regular diet reveals the nutrient gaps. One of the simplest tools to use is the Healthy Diet Pyramid (page 158). Focus on eating food from all the four food groups, each in the right amounts. Eat fresh, wholesome food such as wholegrains, fruit, vegetables, meat and milk products.

(page 158)

Folic Acid in Fortified Food

Folic acid in fortified food is approximately 1.7 times more bioavailable than folate found in food.

Star Nutrients to Focus On

Folic Acid

Folic acid is one of the B-vitamins that is needed for DNA synthesis and cell division, both mechanisms that will step up as soon as you conceive. It is important to consume enough before and during pregnancy as folic acid has been shown to protect against neural tube defects (NTDs).

If you are contemplating pregnancy, the current recommended daily intake of folic acid is 400 mcg a day. You can get more folic acid by eating folate-rich food or taking folic acid, a synthetic compound available through fortified food and supplements.

* Legumes, green leafy vegetables, citrus fruit and juices, and fortified ready-to-eat cereals are good sources.

* Supplementing dietary intake with folic acid has been recommended by many professional organisations because of the difficulty in obtaining the extra folate required through diet alone.

Choline

If you are planning for pregnancy, you require 425 mg of choline daily. Adequate intake of this unique B-vitamin has been found to be associated with a reduced risk of NTDs.

Good sources of choline are egg yolk, beef and baked beans. Fair amounts are found in chicken, milk, salmon, cod, cauliflower, spinach and tofu.

Iron

Many young women are iron deficient due to blood loss during menstruation and poor diet. Women with anaemia put their babies at risk of spontaneous prematurity and intrauterine growth restriction.

To put things right, aim for an iron intake of 19 mg a day. Include adequate portions of iron-rich food daily, such as lean meat, poultry, green leafy vegetables and iron-fortified food.

Calcium and Vitamin D

Calcium is well known for its role in bone development and maintenance. Many women do not consume enough calcium each day. If adequate bone has not been developed before pregnancy and insufficient calcium is consumed, the mother's bone is drawn upon to provide for the needs of the growing foetus.

While awaiting the good news of pregnancy, focus on building up your calcium reserves by boosting your dietary intake. Milk and milk products such as yoghurt and cheese are great sources. Fish with edible bones such as sardines and anchovies (*ikan bilis*) as well as tofu and green leafy vegetables are good choices too. The goal to go for is 800 mg per day.

Vitamin D supports calcium absorption and bone mineralisation. The body can manufacture vitamin D if the skin is exposed to sunlight. However, even in tropical countries, many young women are deficient in vitamin D. Fortified food such as milk, orange juice and some breakfast cereals are the better choices. Fatty fish (salmon, mackerel, tuna and sardine), egg yolk and cheese are fair choices.

Essential Fatty Acids, DHA and AA

Essential fatty acids (EFA), linoleic and alpha-linolenic acid as well as arachidonic acid (AA) and docosahexaenoic acid (DHA) form integral parts of cell membranes and the retina.

EFAs cannot be synthesised in the body and must be consumed as part of the regular diet. Essential fatty acids are found in such food as oily fish, flax seeds, walnuts and vegetable oils. While trying to conceive and during pregnancy, eat at least 360 g of fish each week.

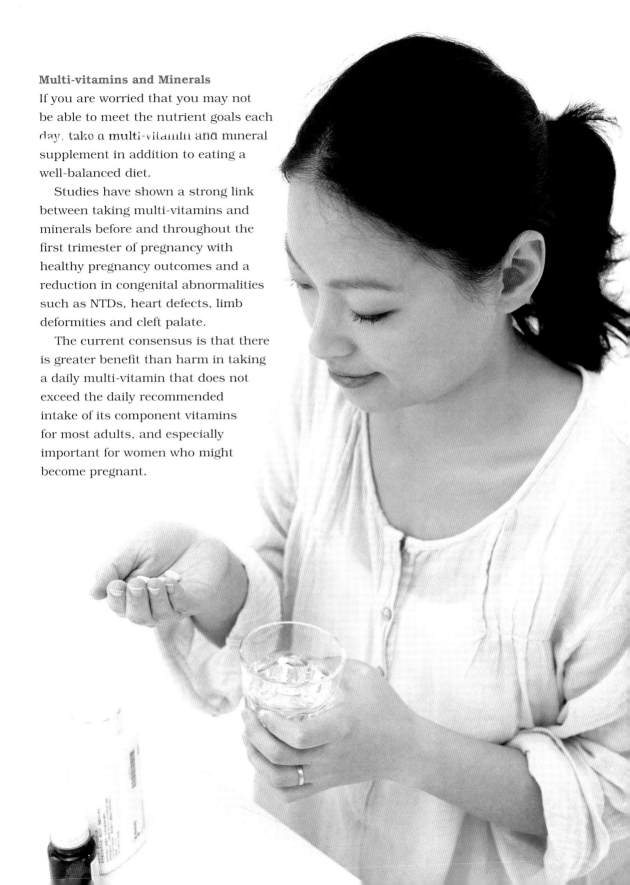

Multi-vitamins and Minerals

If you are worried that you may not be able to meet the nutrient goals each day, take a multi-vitamin and mineral supplement in addition to eating a well-balanced diet.

Studies have shown a strong link between taking multi-vitamins and minerals before and throughout the first trimester of pregnancy with healthy pregnancy outcomes and a reduction in congenital abnormalities such as NTDs, heart defects, limb deformities and cleft palate.

The current consensus is that there is greater benefit than harm in taking a daily multi-vitamin that does not exceed the daily recommended intake of its component vitamins for most adults, and especially important for women who might become pregnant.

Fertility Issues

Many couples conceive almost as soon as they start trying but some are not so fortunate. In fact, one out of five married couples in Singapore has problems trying to conceive.

Common Causes of Infertility

Medical Factors

For females, it may be problems with ovulation. Some do not ovulate or have irregular menstrual cycles where ovulation is unpredictable.

Another common problem is endometriosis where there is a back flow of menstrual blood into the pelvis. This causes scarring of the ovaries and fallopian tubes, leading to impaired fertility.

Pelvic infection, usually the result of an STD, causes blockage of the fallopian tubes, making it difficult for the egg to be fertilised.

For men, the most common problem is sperm dysfunction with low sperm count. In cases where there is no sperm production or where the ducts are blocked, pregnancy will be difficult to achieve.

Age

Fertility declines with age. The biological clock in both men and women ticks away every day. An infant girl has about a million eggs at birth and this declines to about 40,000 when she reaches puberty. The optimal age for conception is between 22 and 26 years of age. The ability to conceive is reduced after the age of 30. It dips by half after the age of 35 and by another half every subsequent five years. Male fertility declines after the age of 40 as the quantity and quality of sperm deteriorate.

Couples over 35 years of age who have had regular unprotected sex for six months without conceiving should seek medical advice as soon as possible.

Body Weight

For women, being overweight or underweight may affect ovulation. Women who are overweight tend to have more complications during pregnancy and birth, such as diabetes and high blood pressure. Underweight women, on the other hand, tend to deliver low birth weight babies.

For men, being overweight is associated with erectile dysfunction, which may affect fertility by reducing the frequency of sexual intimacy.

Timing

The timing for the sperm and egg to meet is also critical. The best days to procreate are likely to be 12 to 16 days into a woman's menstrual cycle when ovulation is expected to occur.

Lifestyle

Smoking, drinking alcohol and taking drugs affect fertility. These toxic substances can cause the menstrual cycle to be irregular and can also affect the quality and quantity of sperm. The risk of miscarriages and having abnormal babies is also increased.

STDs such as chlamydia, gonorrhoea and syphilis cause infertility by damaging the reproductive system.

For men, enjoying saunas and hot baths, and exposure to hot environments or toxic chemicals, such as pesticides, can also cause malfunction of sperm.

Stress

Stress can also lead to infertility. In women, the menstruation cycle can become irregular or absent. In men, it can lead to erectile dysfunction as well as low and malfunctioning sperm. Stress also suppresses sexual desire, thereby reducing the frequency of sexual intercourse.

Diet

Food and fertility are linked. A balanced diet with optimal amounts of energy, protein, vitamins and minerals will improve a couple's chances of conceiving and having a healthy baby.

Enhance Your Fertility

- Reduce stress. Rest and recreation are important when trying to conceive.
- Cut down on cigarettes and alcohol and avoid illicit drugs.
- Maintain a healthy body weight with regular exercise and a well-balanced diet.
- For men, wearing loose underwear and having cold showers may help improve sperm quality.

The First Trimester

Are you pregnant? Although the proof is in the pregnancy test, many women intuitively know that they are, some even before they miss their menstrual period. Some begin to feel symptoms like nausea, aversion to certain smells, sore breasts, larger breasts, fainting and fatigue a week after conception.

Changes to Your Body

You will begin to notice changes in your body due to increased hormone production. Tender breasts, mood swings and tiredness are a few of the changes as your body prepares to support the pregnancy. It is an exhilarating time as you approach this major milestone in your life.

Tender Breasts

Your breasts will feel fuller, heavier and become more sensitive, the areola (the area around the nipple) gets darker. Wearing a comfortable support bra or sports bra will help alleviate some soreness.

Nausea and Vomiting

Many women experience nausea and/or vomiting in early pregnancy. Nausea tends to be worse in the morning but for some women, it can be in the evening or last all day. You may also notice a change in your sense of taste and smell; and you may develop an aversion to certain types of food. The following tips may help.

* Have smaller meals instead of a large one.

* Quell the nausea with dry snacks like sour plums.

* Have a piece of dry toast or a cream cracker before getting out of bed in the morning.

* Drink plenty of fluid (water or fruit juices) in small quantities to avoid dehydration.

* Ginger is a natural remedy for nausea. Try adding it to your cooking.

* Low-fat milk or yoghurt may lower the acidity of the stomach contents, so try consuming some in the morning.

* Avoid eating fried, oily, fatty and spicy food.

* Avoid trigger factors such as noise, jerky movements, smells or odours of food.

* Get enough rest so you wake up in a relaxed mental state.

* Wear motion sickness bands on your wrists. This is based on the principle of acupressure.

* For very severe cases of nausea and vomiting, talk to your doctor about hypnosis.

Fatigue

You will get tired easily as your body prepares to support the pregnancy. Your heart pumps faster and harder, your pulse quickens and your breathing increases. Try to get as much rest as you can.

Frequent Urination

You may urinate more often because during pregnancy, the volume of blood in your body increases, causing more fluid to be processed. As your uterus grows, it will also press on your bladder. The same pressure may cause you to leak urine when sneezing, coughing or laughing. If you are losing sleep due to frequent trips to the bathroom, drink less before going to bed. Avoid drinks that contain caffeine, such as coffee, tea and cola, as these can cause you to urinate more.

Let your doctor know if you feel pain or a burning sensation during urination, or if there is blood in your urine. This may be a sign of a urinary tract infection (UTI). To prevent this, drink plenty of water during the day and go to the bathroom whenever you feel the urge.

Heartburn

During pregnancy, the placenta produces the hormone progesterone, which relaxes the muscles of the valve that separates the oesophagus (the tube that carries food from the throat to the stomach) from the stomach. This allows gastric acids to seep back up the oesophagus, causing an uncomfortable burning sensation known as heartburn. To prevent heartburn, drink plenty of water and eat small, frequent meals. Avoid fried food, carbonated drinks, citrus fruit or juices and spicy food.

A Good Support Bra

Maternity bras are specially designed to support your breasts as they grow bigger and heavier during pregnancy. They will also help you with your posture during the third trimester when your back starts to hurt from carrying the extra weight. When choosing a maternity bra, bear these points in mind:

• Soft bras offer better fit, comfort and support as your breasts change throughout your pregnancy.

• Bras with wider straps provide greater support.

• Bras with wider straps are more comfortable because they will not cut into your shoulders.

• Bras with full cups will provide more comfort and better support.

• Underwire bras can become uncomfortable when your breasts become fuller.

• Bras with front fasteners may be more convenient.

Constipation

Your stomach and intestines take longer to empty their contents due to hormonal changes, thus leading to constipation. To maintain regular bowel movement, eat plenty of wholegrain food, fruit and vegetables, and drink lots of fluid. Regular physical activity may help. Talk to your doctor if your constipation persists.

Dizziness

Changes in blood circulation may make you feel a little dizzy. Stress, fatigue and hunger may make you feel worse. Avoid prolonged standing. Lie down and rest should you feel dizzy. When you need to get up from a sitting or lying down position, do so slowly, as any sudden movements may cause your blood pressure to drop.

See your obstetrician immediately if you have severe dizziness accompanied by abdominal pain or vaginal bleeding. This may be an early sign of an ectopic pregnancy—a condition in which the fertilised egg is implanted outside the uterus. This can be life-threatening as it may cause internal bleeding.

Emotional Changes

While you may be happily looking forward to having your baby, you may also feel anxious and sometimes depressed. It is natural to feel some anxiety about your baby's health, your adjustment to becoming a mother, the financial demands and the responsibilities that come with raising a child. You will wonder how this will affect your relationship with your spouse and whether you will be a good parent. If you are working, you may worry about balancing the demands of family and career. These feelings are normal. Share your feelings with your spouse, other close family members and friends to get support and encouragement.

Your Baby's Development

Weeks 1 to 4

Life begins when a sperm penetrates the outer wall of an egg and fuses with it. This takes place in the fallopian tube. The fertilised egg then moves down towards the womb and, within a few days, multiplies itself into a cluster of cells called the blastocyst. The inner group of cells develops into the baby while the outer group becomes the membranes (amniotic sac) in which the baby develops and the placenta which sticks to the wall of the uterus by a process called implantation. The placenta starts to nourish and protect the developing baby.

Weeks 5 to 8

Your baby's head, heart, limbs and spinal cord begin to form. By the eighth week, the baby has a recognisable human form with developing limbs.

Weeks 9 to 12

The baby has a small body dominated by a large head as the brain and head grow more rapidly than the rest of the body. The vital organs—brain, lungs, liver, kidneys and intestines—are formed and functional. The heart starts to pump blood to all parts of the body.

First Trimester Screening

This prenatal test offers early information about the baby's health. It is done between weeks 11 and 14 of pregnancy. First trimester screening poses no risk of miscarriage.

Blood Test and Nuchal Translucency Ultrasound Scan

There are two components to this test: a blood test to measure levels of two pregnancy-specific substances and a specialised ultrasound examination (Nuchal Translucency Ultrasound Scan) to measure the baby's nuchal fold, which is a specific area at the back of the neck. The measurement indicates the risk of Down syndrome. The thicker the nuchal fold, the greater the risk.

Using your age and the results of the blood test and ultrasound, your obstetrician will be able to gauge your risk of carrying a baby with Down syndrome or Edwards syndrome. Both conditions cause mental retardation.

The results are given as a probability. It correctly identifies about 85 percent of women who are carrying a baby with Down syndrome. About 5 percent of women have a false-positive result, meaning that the test result is positive but the baby does not actually have Down syndrome. Generally, if the risk is one in 250 or higher, the test is considered positive.

If your risk level is low, first trimester screening can offer reassurance of a healthy pregnancy. If your risk level is moderate or high, you may choose to do more invasive diagnostic testing, such as Chorionic Villus Sampling (CVS) or amniocentesis (pages 40–41).

Because first trimester screening can be done earlier than most other prenatal screening tests, you will have the results early in your pregnancy. This will give you more time to make decisions about further diagnostic tests, medical treatment and the course of your pregnancy. If your baby is diagnosed with a genetic condition, you will also have more time to prepare for the possibility of caring for a child with special needs.

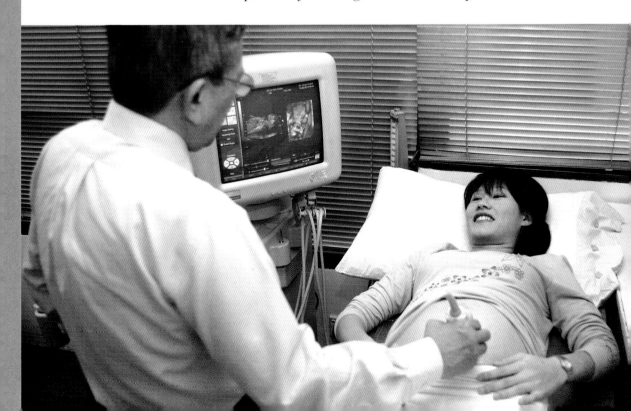

GESTATIONAL DIABETES

Some women develop diabetes when they are pregnant. This is known as gestational diabetes. In gestational diabetes, the pregnant woman's blood sugar level is raised but will return to normal after delivery.

Risk Factors for Gestational Diabetes

☐ Family history of diabetes.

☐ History of repeated miscarriages or stillbirths.

☐ Overweight or excessive weight gain during pregnancy.

☐ The unborn baby is large.

☐ Twin pregnancy.

Effects on Mother and Baby

High blood sugar can be harmful to both mother and baby. Left uncontrolled, it may lead to urinary and vaginal infections as well as hypertension during pregnancy. It can also lead to miscarriage, stillbirth and premature birth. The delivery may be more difficult and chances of having a caesarean-section are higher.

After delivery, the baby may suffer from low blood sugar levels and jaundice, and may have breathing difficulties. When the baby grows up, he is also more likely to be obese or may develop diabetes later in life.

Treatment

If you suffer from gestational diabetes, your obstetrician will refer you to a dietitian who will have you follow a diabetic diet. If your blood sugar cannot be controlled by diet, insulin injections may be prescribed.

The Second Trimester

Shopping for maternity clothes is just one of the many enjoyable aspects of being pregnant! Here are some tips to help you find attractive yet comfortable maternity clothes as your body changes and your baby bump starts to show.

- Look into your wardrobe (or your spouse's!) and you may find some bigger size clothes that you can wear at least for the earlier part of your pregnancy.

- Go for separate tops and bottoms so you can mix and match for different looks.

- For skirts or trousers, look for drawstrings and adjustable waistbands as these offer comfort and fit as your shape changes.

- Select clothes in stretchy fabric as these will expand as you expand.

- Choose clothes made of natural fibres like cotton and silk to keep you cool and comfortable.

Changes to Your Body

You will feel a renewed sense of well-being and be more energetic in the second trimester. Your baby bump will start to show, and people will begin noticing. As your baby develops, you will also start to feel him moving in your womb.

There will be more changes to your body as your pregnancy progresses. Enjoy this second trimester and spend as much time as possible with your spouse and other family members while you still have the opportunity. Use this time to plan and prepare for the arrival of your baby as well.

Larger Breasts

Stimulated by oestrogen and progesterone, your breasts grow larger during the second trimester. Additional fat may also accumulate in your breasts. It is advisable that you wear a support bra at this stage.

Braxton Hicks Contractions

Your uterus may start contracting, and you may experience with uncomfortable but painless Braxton Hicks contractions in your lower abdomen. These contractions are usually weak, and they come and go unpredictably. Some women do not even notice them but should they get uncomfortable for you, changing your position and deep, rhythmic breathing can help alleviate the discomfort.

Darker Skin and Stretch Marks

Certain parts of your face, nipples and the line that runs from your umbilicus to your lower abdomen may become darker.

You may also notice pink, red or purple stretch marks along your abdomen, breasts, upper arms, buttocks or thighs. These stretch marks may cause you to itch, so moisturise well to soothe the discomfort. The stretch marks will fade in intensity over time.

Gum Problems

Hormonal changes and increased blood volume circulating throughout your body may cause your gums to become hypersensitive, and they may become inflamed and bleed when you brush your teeth. To overcome this, switch to a softer toothbrush.

Nasal Problems

Pregnancy hormones may cause the lining of your nose and sinuses to swell, making it feel as though your nose is perpetually blocked and stuffy. These hormones may also cause the tiny blood vessels in your nose to dilate which may, in turn, cause nosebleeds, especially if you blow your nose too hard.

Leg Cramps

Your expanding uterus may put pressure on the blood vessels in your legs, causing leg cramps. Leg cramps can occur at any time, but you will feel them mostly at bedtime. To relieve leg cramp, stretch the affected calf muscle by flexing your toes back towards your shin.

Fatigue

Although you may not feel as tired as you did in the first trimester, it is still important that you get enough rest. It is better to take frequent rest periods than wait until you are really tired.

Bladder and Kidney Infections

Hormonal changes slow the flow of urine, and your expanding uterus may get in the way of the flow, increasing the risk of bladder and kidney infections. Left untreated, urinary infections increase the risk of preterm labour. Let your obstetrician know if you feel pain or a burning sensation during urination, or if there is blood in your urine, so any infection can be treated head on.

Emotional Changes

As your pregnancy progresses, changes in your body's shape and function may affect your emotions. Some women feel a heightened sexuality during pregnancy. Others feel unattractive, especially as their bellies grow. If you are struggling with your body image, share your concerns with your spouse. Express love and affection in ways that help you feel most comfortable.

It is also important to remember that your spouse may also be experiencing emotional changes at this time. Impending fatherhood may bring on feelings of fear and anticipation. Talk openly about what you are both going through and support each other.

Your Baby's Development

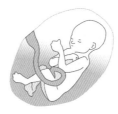

Weeks 13 to 16

Your baby's circulatory system and urinary tract are working well. He can grasp, squint, frown and grimace. His fingernails are fully formed. He can flex his joints and limbs. You may be able to tell the sex of your baby through an ultrasound scan.

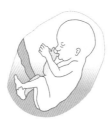

Weeks 17 to 20

Your baby is completely covered with fine, soft hair called lanugo. The lanugo helps hold the vernix caseosa, a greasy, cheese-like coating that protects his delicate skin. Your baby's bones start to develop. Small bones in the ear harden by week 18 and he can hear your heart beating, your stomach rumbling and may even be startled by loud noises in your surroundings! If you talk, read or sing to your baby, he may react to the sound by kicking. You may start to discern his movements, called quickening, at this time.

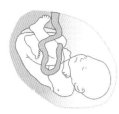

Weeks 21 to 24

The testes begin to descend from the abdomen in baby boys, and the uterus and ovaries are in place, complete with a lifetime supply of eggs, in baby girls.

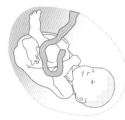

Weeks 25 to 28

His organs are mostly developed and his brain development speeds up. He can open and shut his eyes. His kicking becomes stronger.

Second Trimester Screening

Triple Test

Between weeks 15 and 20, you might be offered the Triple Test, also known as the multiple marker screening. This is a blood test that measures three substances to evaluate your risk of carrying a baby who has Down syndrome, Edwards syndrome or spinal defects.

Second Trimester Ultrasound Assessment

A detailed ultrasound assessment (Foetal Anomaly Scan) can be done between weeks 18 and 20 of pregnancy. At this stage, parts of the baby's body can be seen clearly.

During the scan, your obstetrician will examine each part of the baby, determine the position of the placenta, assess the amount of amniotic fluid and measure the growth. Special attention is paid to the brain, face, spine, heart, stomach, bowel, kidneys and limbs.

In women at high risk of preterm delivery (those who have had multiple pregnancies, previous preterm birth(s), abnormalities of the uterus or cervical surgery), the obstetrician may do a transvaginal scan to measure the length of the cervix. This scan checks for early signs of the cervix opening before the baby is due.

PREECLAMPSIA

Preeclampsia is a condition in which a pregnant woman suddenly has high blood pressure and excess protein in her urine. This condition usually develops after 20 weeks of pregnancy. Left untreated, preeclampsia can lead to serious —even fatal—complications for both mother and baby. The other signs of preeclampsia are:

☐ Severe headaches.

☐ Changes in vision, including temporary loss of vision, blurred vision or sensitivity to light.

☐ Upper abdominal pain, usually under your ribs on the right side.

☐ Nausea or vomiting.

☐ Dizziness.

☐ Decreased urine output.

☐ Sudden weight gain, typically more than 1 kg a week.

☐ Swelling in the face and hands.

Because headaches, nausea, and aches and pains are common pregnancy complaints, it is difficult to know if the symptoms are simply part of being pregnant or if they indicate a serious problem—especially if it is your first pregnancy. To play it safe, check with your doctor. You are at higher risk of preeclampsia if you are:

☐ A first-time mother.

☐ Diabetic.

☐ Obese.

☐ Carrying more than one baby.

☐ Suffering from high blood pressure, autoimmune disease or kidney disease prior to pregnancy.

Complications of Preeclampsia

☐ Decreased blood flow to the placenta. This reduces the baby's oxygen supply and nutrients, potentially slowing the baby's growth and increasing the risk of a low birth weight infant and may be life-threatening.

☐ Placental abruption. The placenta prematurely separates from the uterus causing sudden deprivation of oxygen to the baby. The mother may also experience heavy bleeding.

☐ Premature delivery. Sometimes, early delivery is needed to prevent potentially life-threatening complications such as eclamptic seizures, stroke, heart, liver and kidney failure.

☐ Future cardiovascular disease. The mother may be at increased risk of cardiovascular disease later in life, although her blood pressure may return to normal after delivery.

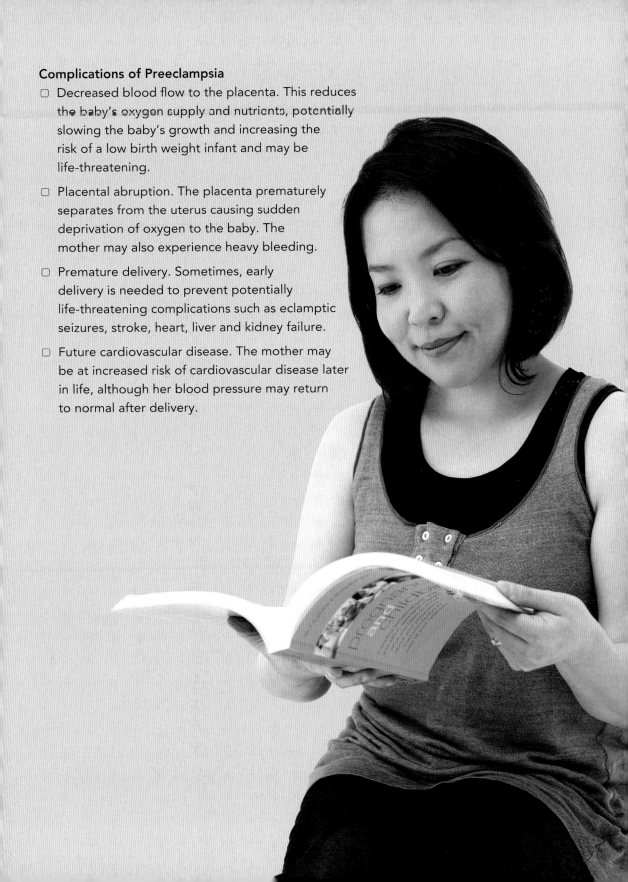

The Third Trimester

Changes to Your Body

The third trimester can be physically and emotionally challenging, but also the most exciting as you eagerly anticipate the birth of your baby.

While you were more energetic in the second trimester, you will begin to slow down in the third trimester as your baby grows larger. Listen to your body and rest when you need to.

Backache

Pregnancy hormones relax the joints between the bones in your pelvis and spine. Bad posture, which is common in pregnancy, may aggravate backache. To ease the pain, sit in chairs with good back support. Apply a heating pad or ice pack to the painful area. Ask your spouse for a massage. Wear low-heeled shoes with good arch support.

Shortness of Breath

You may feel breathless as your womb expands and pushes up your lungs. Practise good posture and sleep with your upper body propped up on pillows to relieve pressure on your lungs. Aerobic exercises can help.

Heartburn

Although you may have experienced this symptom in the first trimester, heartburn is more common in the last trimester when the growing uterus pushes your stomach upwards. The following tips may help.

* Sleep propped up with pillows. Gravity will help your stomach acids flow down.

* Avoid consuming carbonated drinks, alcohol, caffeine, chocolate, citrus fruit and juices, vinegar, and spicy, fried and oily food.

* Eat small meals. Take time to eat and chew thoroughly. Do not lie down immediately after a meal. Try to sit up for at least 20 minutes after eating.

* Do not eat too close to bedtime. Try to eat at least two to three hours before bedtime.

* Drink plenty of fluid in small quantities between meals.

* Wear loose, comfortable clothing; avoid any tightness around your waist and tummy.

* If these solutions do not work, talk to your doctor who may prescribe antacids.

Spider Veins, Varicose Veins and Haemorrhoids

Increased blood circulation may cause small reddish spots that sprout tiny blood vessels on your face, neck and/or arms. Blue or reddish lines beneath the surface of the skin (varicose veins) may also appear, particularly in the legs. Varicose veins in your rectum (haemorrhoids) may occur.

If you have painful varicose veins, wear support stockings and elevate your legs while seated or lying down.

To prevent haemorrhoids, avoid constipation. Include more fibre in your diet and drink more fluids.

Production of Colostrum

As delivery approaches, your nipples may start leaking colostrum—the yellowish fluid that will nourish your baby during the first few days of life. There will only be a few drops, if any, but should you feel uncomfortable with the dampness, insert a nursing pad into your bra.

Frequent Urination

As your baby moves deeper into your pelvis, you will feel more pressure on your bladder. You may find yourself urinating more often, especially during the night.

Braxton Hicks Contractions

These contractions may occur more frequently as your body prepares for the impending birth of your baby. Practise deep breathing to relieve the discomfort.

Vaginal Discharge

Heavy vaginal discharge is common but you may be screened for Group B Streptococcus (GBS). This is a common bacterium that is usually harmless in adults but babies who get infected can become critically ill. If a swab from your vagina tests positive for GBS, you will probably be given intravenous antibiotics during labour.

Swelling

As your growing uterus puts pressure on the veins that return blood from your feet and legs, you may notice your feet and ankles becoming swollen. At the same time, hormonal changes may cause water retention, leaving your face and eyelids puffy in the mornings.

To reduce swelling of the feet, use cold compresses on the affected areas. Lie down and rest or elevate your feet and legs with pillows while you sleep. Swimming may also help.

Emotional Changes

As anticipation grows, you may have feelings of apprehension and fear about childbirth. Talk with friends who have had positive birth experiences and get support and encouragement from them.

The reality of parenthood is fast approaching and you may feel anxious and overwhelmed, especially if this is your first baby. You will feel less stressed and more positive if you take this time to make sure that you have everything ready for the arrival of your baby.

Your Baby's Development

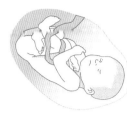

Weeks 29 to 32
Your baby's skeleton hardens and his brain, muscles, lungs and digestive tract continue to mature. His head grows to accommodate the expansion of his brain. His limbs fill out and he will not move as much.

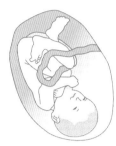

Weeks 33 to 36
Your baby's brain continues to grow rapidly. More fat accumulates under his skin, which will help to regulate his body temperature after birth. He will turn upside down into the position for delivery.

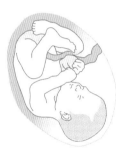

Weeks 37 to 40
The baby is now fully formed with the head more in proportion with the body. He gains weight slowly but steadily in preparation for birth. His lungs mature and a hormone in his lungs is released to trigger contractions.

Prenatal Testing

Prenatal testing includes a battery of tests to assess diseases or conditions in your unborn baby. There is no test that can guarantee a healthy baby but prenatal testing can detect neural tube defects such as spina bifida, chromosomal abnormalities like Down syndrome and other conditions like cleft palate.

Screening Tests

Screening tests are done to identify whether your baby is more likely to have certain conditions but these tests cannot make a definitive diagnosis. Screening tests pose no risk for you or your baby.

Diagnostic Tests

If a screening test indicates a possible problem, you may consider doing an invasive prenatal diagnostic test, such as Chorionic Villus Sampling (CVS) or amniocentesis (pages 40–41). It is important to make an informed decision about prenatal testing, especially if you are screening for foetal conditions that cannot be treated. Here is a list of things you should think about as you decide whether or not to go for a diagnostic test.

What are the risks?
Weigh the risks of specific prenatal tests, such as anxiety, pain or possible miscarriage, against the value of knowing the results.

How accurate are the results?
Prenatal testing is not perfect. The proportion of false-negative and false-positive results varies from test to test.

What will you do with the test results?
Normal results can ease your anxiety but if prenatal testing indicates that the baby may have a birth defect, you may be faced with heart-wrenching decisions, such as whether to continue with the pregnancy or abort it. On the other hand, it gives you the opportunity to plan for your baby's care in advance.

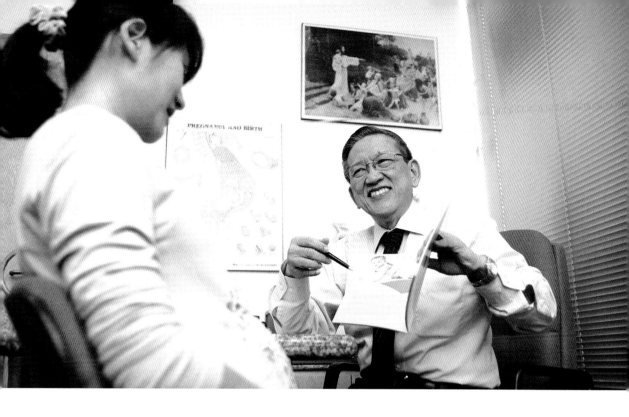

Will the results affect your prenatal care?

Some tests detect problems that can be treated while you are pregnant. In other cases, prenatal testing alerts your obstetrician to a condition that requires immediate treatment after birth.

Prenatal Testing at a Glance

Trimester	Screening Test	Diagnostic Test
First Trimester (Weeks 1 to 13)	**Nuchal Translucency Ultrasound Scan** • Tests for Down syndrome and Edwards syndrome • Done between weeks 11 and 14 of pregnancy	**Chorionic Villus Sampling (CVS)** • Tests for chromosomal abnormalities and cystic fibrosis • Done between weeks 10 and 12 of pregnancy
Second Trimester (Weeks 14 to 28)	**Triple Test Ultrasound** • Tests for Down syndrome, Edwards syndrome and spinal defects • Done between weeks 15 and 20 of pregnancy	**Amniocentesis** • Tests for chromosomal problems and foetal infections • Done between weeks 16 and 20 of pregnancy
Third Trimester (Weeks 29 to 40)	Nil	Nil

CHORIONIC VILLUS SAMPLING

During pregnancy, the placenta provides oxygen and nutrients to the baby and removes the baby's waste products. The chorionic villi are finger-like projections that make up most of the placenta and share the baby's genetic makeup.

Chorionic Villus Sampling (CVS) is a prenatal test in which a tiny piece of placenta (chorionic villi) is removed for testing. It can reveal whether the baby has a chromosomal abnormality. It is usually done between weeks 10 and 12 of pregnancy. CVS can also be used to diagnose other genetic disorders such as cystic fibrosis.

When to Consider CVS

☐ If the results from a prenatal screening test is abnormal. CVS will confirm or rule out a diagnosis.

☐ If there was a chromosomal abnormality in a previous pregnancy.

☐ If you are aged 35 or older. Babies born to women aged 35 and above have a higher risk of chromosomal abnormalities.

☐ If you or your spouse is a known carrier of a genetic disorder, or there is a family history of a specific genetic disorder.

Some of the Risks of CVS

☐ Overall, CVS has a one in 100 risk of miscarriage. The risk appears to be slightly higher when the tissue sample is taken through the cervix (transcervical) rather than the abdominal wall (transabdominal). The risk of miscarriage also increases if the baby is smaller than normal for his gestational age.

☐ You may feel cramping after the test. Vaginal bleeding is also possible, especially if the sample is taken through your cervix rather than the abdominal wall.

☐ It may cause some of the baby's blood cells to enter your bloodstream. If you have Rh negative blood, you will be given a drug called Rh immunoglobulin after the test to prevent your body from producing antibodies against your baby's blood cells.

- Although very rare, CVS may trigger a uterine infection.

- Some studies suggest that CVS may cause defects in a baby's fingers or toes. However, the risk appears to increase if it is done before the ninth week of pregnancy.

- There is a rare chance of a false-positive test, meaning that the test is positive but no disease exists.

AMNIOCENTESIS

Amniocentesis is a specialised diagnostic test usually performed in the second trimester between weeks 16 and 20 of pregnancy. It is used for the diagnosis of chromosomal problems and foetal infections, and involves taking a sample of amniotic fluid from your uterus. By the second trimester, there is enough amniotic fluid surrounding the baby for the doctor to take an adequate sample without putting the baby at risk. Guided by ultrasound, your obstetrician will insert a long thin needle through your abdominal wall into your uterus, taking care to avoid the placenta and the baby.

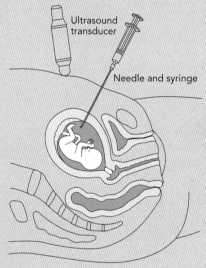

Ultrasound transducer

Needle and syringe

Some of the Risks of Amniocentesis

- Early amniocentesis carries a slight risk of miscarriage often due to the rupture of the amniotic sac. The risk of miscarriage is highest when the procedure is done early in pregnancy.

- Cramping is possible after amniocentesis. Some women experience a small amount of vaginal bleeding.

- During amniocentesis, the baby may move an arm or leg into the path of the needle but serious needle injuries are rare.

- There is a very small chance that amniotic fluid may leak through the vagina after amniocentesis. If the leak is sealed, the pregnancy may proceed normally.

- Although rare, amniocentesis may cause the baby's blood cells to enter the mother's bloodstream. If you have Rh negative blood, you will be given a drug called Rh immunoglobulin after amniocentesis to prevent your body from producing antibodies against your baby's blood cells.

- Very rarely, amniocentesis may trigger a uterine infection.

TWIN PREGNANCY

Twins can be non-identical (80 percent of all twin births) or identical (20 percent of all twin births). Non-identical twins occur when two separate eggs are fertilised by two different sperms. Each twin has his own placenta and amniotic sac.

Identical twins occur when a single fertilised egg splits and develops into two babies. Identical twins may share a placenta but each baby usually has a separate amniotic sac. Genetically, the two babies are identical. They will be of the same sex and look exactly alike. Rarely, identical twins fail to completely separate into two individuals and become conjoined twins (Siamese twins).

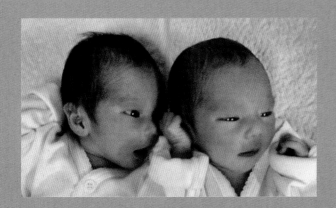

A twin pregnancy is more likely to occur if there is a history of twins in the family, if the woman conceives after the age of 35 or had assisted reproductive technologies such as In-Vitro Fertilisation (IVF) or Intracytoplasmic Sperm Injection (ICSI).

Diagnosis

Your obstetrician may suspect a twin pregnancy if your uterus is larger than normal. This will be confirmed by an ultrasound test. Sometimes, a seemingly normal twin pregnancy is later found to have only a single baby. This is known as the vanishing twin syndrome. There is often no clear explanation for the loss.

What To Expect during a Twin Pregnancy

☐ More frequent checkups. You will see your obstetrician more often to track your babies' growth and development, monitor your health and watch for signs of preterm labour. You may need frequent ultrasound scans or other tests.

- More emphasis on certain nutrients. You will need more folic acid, calcium, iron, protein and other essential nutrients.

- More weight gain. The recommendation is about 16 to 20 kg for women carrying twins who had a healthy weight before pregnancy.

- More precautions. Your obstetrician may ask you to limit some of your activities such as work, travel and exercise as your pregnancy progresses. Although bed rest has not been proven as an effective way to prevent preterm labour, it is sometimes suggested when the mother's blood pressure is high or when there is concern about the babies' growth.

Possible Complications of Twin Pregnancies

- High blood pressure. High blood pressure during a twin pregnancy is more likely. When high blood pressure is accompanied by protein in the urine, the condition is known as preeclampsia (pages 32–33). Careful management is needed to prevent serious complications in both mother and babies.

- Preterm birth. If you have signs of preterm labour, you may be given steroid injections to speed up your babies' lung development. Premature babies may have low birth weights, breathing and digestive difficulties, under-developed organs, learning disabilities and developmental problems.

- Delayed-interval delivery. This refers to the rare situation when one baby is delivered prematurely while the other baby is able to continue developing in the womb.

- Twin-twin transfusion. With identical twins, it is possible for the babies to share the placenta unequally. This causes one baby to receive too much blood and the other too little. This is a serious complication for both babies that may require aggressive intervention during pregnancy.

- Caesarean-section delivery. Caesarean-section deliveries are common for twin pregnancies, especially if the babies are not in a head-down position. In some cases, complications after the vaginal delivery of the first twin may result in a caesarean-section delivery for the second twin.

Nutrition during Pregnancy

One of the first few things you should think about once you know you are pregnant is how much you need to eat to support your growing baby. Read on to know what, when and how much you need to eat to nourish a pregnancy.

First Trimester

At this stage, the foetus does not increase very much in weight or size, so your energy needs do not increase substantially. But the need for vitamins, minerals and protein increases to support rapid cell division and organ development in the foetus.

So, you really do not have to eat a lot more at this point but focus on selecting nutrient-dense food including a maternal milk supplement to deliver valuable nutrients such as protein, vitamins and minerals.

Second and Third Trimesters

Your caloric needs increase in the second and third trimesters as the foetus gains weight rapidly. In the last three months of pregnancy, the foetus triples in weight and deposits large amounts of nutrients. For example, DHA accumulates in the eyes, brain and nervous system; iron is packed away in the liver for the first six months of life, when breastfeeding is exclusive; and calcium is deposited to strengthen bones. In addition, your body changes to support the pregnancy.

Your caloric needs will increase from between 340 kcal each day in the second trimester to about 450 kcal per day in the third trimester. Aim to eat enough—not too little and not too much—and enjoy a wide variety of nourishing food.

Add Value

Eat a Well-balanced Diet
Include a variety of nutritious food such as wholegrain bread, brown rice, fruit, vegetables, legumes, lean meat, fish,

poultry, eggs, nuts, seeds and low fat dairy products such as milk, yoghurt and cheese in your diet each day.

Choose Low Fat Food

While fat is an essential nutrient at this time, lower fat food choices will help you achieve appropriate weight gain, so you do not have to deal with losing the excessive weight gained.

Add DHA

DHA accumulates rapidly in the brain and eyes of your baby during the last trimester and through the first two years of life. Current recommendations support an intake of 200 mg per day throughout pregnancy. Anchovies, salmon, sardines, tuna, mackerel and maternal milk supplements are great sources of this beneficial nutrient.

Meet Your Folic Acid Needs

Folic acid helps cells multiply, a process critical to healthy baby development. Aim for an intake of 600 mcg per day. Folic acid is found in leafy green vegetables like spinach, melons, oranges and fortified food. Your doctor might recommend that you take supplements to meet the increased need for folic acid.

Include Choline

Another B-vitamin, choline helps prevent NTDs. In the growing foetus, choline is involved in the development of the hippocampus, which is known to be the seat of memory in the brain. The goal is to aim for 450 mg per day. Choline is found in eggs, beef, chicken, turkey, salmon and baked beans.

Consume More B-Complex Vitamins

Working together, these water soluble nutrients support metabolism, promote cell growth and division, maintain healthy skin and muscle tone, and enhance immune and nervous system functions. Wholegrains, fruit, vegetables, meat, poultry, fish, milk and legumes are excellent sources of many B-vitamins.

Vital Nutrients during Pregnancy

- Protein is needed to build muscle and tissue and form the placenta.
- Folic acid is critical for cell division and organ formation.
- Iron helps make new red blood cells.
- Zinc assists with growth and development.

Incorporate Iron

Iron helps build red blood cells and prevent anaemia. Iron supports the expansion of your blood volume and baby's brain growth, development of the nervous system and neurotransmitters.

Lack of iron during baby's development can negatively impact learning and behaviour. Iron is essential to build up baby's liver stores which will last for the first six months of life. Aim to include about 27 mg in your diet per day. Iron-rich food include lean meat, fish, poultry, legumes and green leafy vegetables.

Concentrate on Calcium

Calcium is needed to help build and strengthen baby's skeleton and teeth. Aim for an intake of about 1000 mg of calcium per day. Include dairy products like milk, yoghurt and cheese in your diet as they are the best sources of calcium. Fish with edible bones, green leafy vegetables, legumes and calcium-fortified food are also good sources.

Understand Your Zinc Needs

Zinc is essential for protein synthesis, integrity of cell membranes, tissue growth and repair, wound healing, bone mineralisation, blood clotting and cognitive functions. Rich sources of zinc are oysters, beef, seafood, poultry, nuts and seeds, wholegrains, tofu and legumes.

Increase Fibre and Fluid Intake

Increase your fibre intake by about 10 percent during pregnancy. Fibre, including fructo-oligosaccharides (FOS), supports bowel regularity and the growth of beneficial bacteria in the gut, improving maternal immunity. Wholegrain bread, fruit, vegetables and legumes are rich sources of fibre. For bowel regularity, increase fluid intake by drinking water, soup, juice and milk.

Manage Discomforts

Morning sickness as well as food cravings and aversions are common pregnancy discomforts that challenge food intake. A well-designed maternal nutritional supplement will help you fill the nutritional gaps in your diet. Select a low fat, nutrient-dense supplement that provides all the nutrients your baby needs for optimal growth, development and health.

Morning Sickness

Although often referred to as morning sickness, many expectant women experience it at other times of the day as well. This discomfort occurs mostly in the first trimester, but some women continue to experience nausea throughout their pregnancies. Eating small frequent meals, having dry toast or a cracker before getting out of bed, eating a small snack before bedtime and avoiding greasy, rich, fatty and spicy food may help alleviate the problem. If these simple steps do not work, talk to your doctor about it.

Heartburn

This burning sensation in the food pipe may be relieved by eating smaller meals, eating slowly and drinking fluid in between meals. Some doctors recommend not bending, stooping or lying down soon after eating a meal.

Indigestion

You may experience increased bloating, belching and nausea. Again, smaller but more frequent meals may help, as will eating slowly and chewing your food well.

Constipation

For bowel regularity, drink plenty of water and eat fibre-rich food such as fruit, vegetables, wholegrains and beans.

Food Cravings and Aversions

Some pregnant women experience an increased preference or dislike for specific food. Should you experience such cravings or aversions, just bear in mind to eat a well-balanced diet overall.

Food to Avoid during Pregnancy

- Raw or undercooked meat and poultry.
- Raw or soft-boiled eggs.
- Untreated goat's milk.
- Soft, ripened cheese, including Brie, feta, Camembert, blue-veined cheese, unpasteurised cheese and cheese made from goat's or sheep's milk.
- Unwashed fruit and vegetables.
- Cooked-chilled ready meals.
- Unheated cooked-chilled meals.
- Pre-cooked and chilled poultry food that may not have been reheated safely.
- Raw or undercooked fish and shellfish in dishes like sashimi and *yu sheng*.
- Large fish, especially swordfish, shark, king mackerel and tilefish.

Exercise during Pregnancy

Exercise can help prevent or reduce discomfort from the extra weight of pregnancy, boost energy levels and improve your overall health. It helps you prepare for labour by increasing your stamina and muscle strength. It may even shorten your labour and speed up your recovery after delivery.

Exercise with Care

If you experience any of the following symptoms while exercising, stop and call your obstetrician immediately.

- Blurred vision
- Dizziness
- Nausea
- Fatigue
- Shortness of breath
- Chest pain
- Abdominal pain
- Vaginal bleeding

Types of Exercises

Most exercises are safe during pregnancy, provided you do them with caution. Swimming, brisk walking, stationary cycling and low-impact aerobics carry little risk of injury and can be done in moderation. You should choose exercises that do not require too much balance or coordination.

If you exercised regularly before pregnancy, you can probably continue to work out at the same level while you are pregnant, as long as you feel comfortable and do not over-strain yourself. If you have not exercised before, start with just 5 minutes of exercise and gradually increase the duration.

Regular exercise can help you cope with the physical changes of pregnancy and build stamina for the challenges ahead. If you have not been exercising regularly, use pregnancy as your motivation to start doing so.

Here are some tips to bear in mind while exercising:

* Wear loose-fitting, comfortable clothes and a good support bra.

* Choose a pair of comfortable shoes.

* Stretch before and after each workout.

* Exercise on a flat, level surface to prevent injury.

* After doing floor exercises, get up slowly and gradually to prevent dizziness.

* Do not exercise until the point of exhaustion.

* Do not exercise in hot and humid weather.

* Drink plenty of water before, during and after your workout.

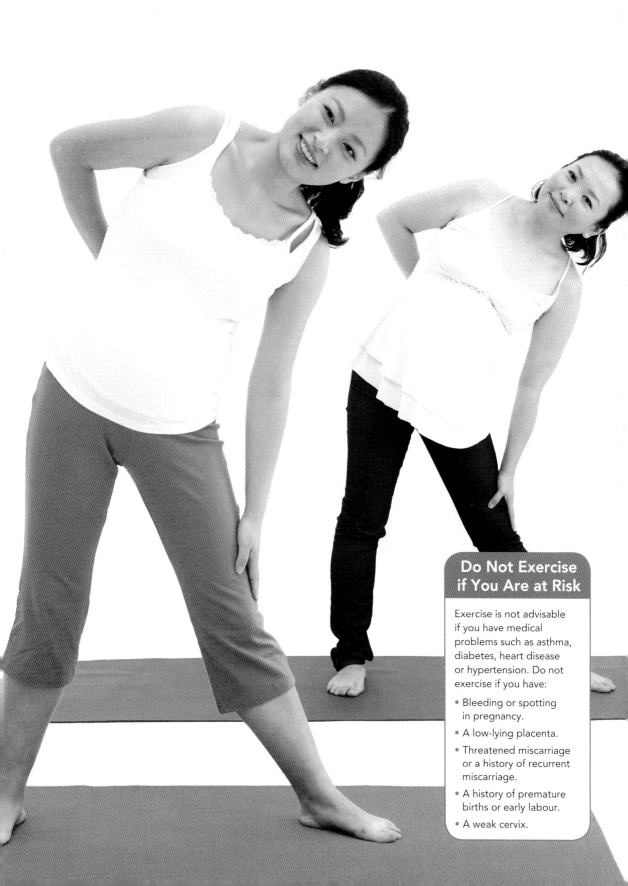

Do Not Exercise if You Are at Risk

Exercise is not advisable if you have medical problems such as asthma, diabetes, heart disease or hypertension. Do not exercise if you have:

- Bleeding or spotting in pregnancy.

- A low-lying placenta.

- Threatened miscarriage or a history of recurrent miscarriage.

- A history of premature births or early labour.

- A weak cervix.

Sex during Pregnancy

Has pregnancy perked up your interest in sexual intercourse? Or is intercourse the last thing on your mind? Sexual desire differs from person to person and it varies at different phases of pregnancy. Having sex during pregnancy is very personal. Share your needs and concerns with your spouse in an open and loving way and make decisions together.

Changes in Sexual Desire

In the first trimester, breast tenderness, nausea, vomiting and fears of miscarriage may sap your sexual desire. During the second trimester, increased blood flow to your sexual organs and breasts may rekindle your desire for sexual intercourse. By the third trimester, fear of premature birth, an enlarged womb, back pain and other symptoms may once again dampen your enthusiasm for intercourse.

The desire for intercourse in your spouse is likely to change as well. Some men feel closer to their wives and enjoy the physical changes in pregnancy. Others may experience decreased desire because of anxiety about the risk of miscarriage and premature birth.

Common Concerns

Is sexual intercourse advisable during pregnancy?

There is no hard and fast rule on sexual intercourse during pregnancy. As long as your pregnancy is proceeding normally, you can continue to have sexual intercourse. You may worry that it will lead to a miscarriage, especially in the first trimester, but miscarriages are usually related to chromosomal abnormalities or other problems in the developing baby and not sexual intercourse.

Will having sexual intercourse harm my baby?

Your developing baby is protected by the amniotic fluid in your uterus as well as the mucous plug that blocks the cervix throughout most of your pregnancy. Sexual activity will not affect your baby unless your spouse is infected with an STD.

Will having an orgasm trigger premature labour?

While orgasms can cause some uterine contractions, these contractions are different from the contractions you will feel during labour and will not increase the risk of premature birth or trigger labour even as your due date approaches.

When to Avoid Sex

Although most women can safely have sexual intercourse throughout pregnancy, your obstetrician may recommend avoiding sex if:

* You have vaginal bleeding.

* You have a history of repeated miscarriages.

* You are at risk of premature labour.

* You are leaking amniotic fluid.

* Your cervix is weak (cervical incompetence).

* Your placenta is low lying (placenta preavia).

Weight Gain during Pregnancy

As your baby bulge begins to show, you will also notice that you are starting to gain weight. While weight gain is important and necessary to help support a healthy pregnancy, be wary of the old adage about eating for two. Gaining too much weight or gaining too little may be harmful for you and your baby.

Monitoring Your Weight Gain

- During the initial prenatal checkups, your doctor will advise you on a healthy pregnancy weight gain plan based on your pre-pregnancy weight.
- Your weight will be recorded and monitored at every prenatal checkup.
- Speak to your doctor should you have concerns about your weight gain.

In the first trimester, the weight gain is small, only 1 to 2 kg. Most weight, about 5 to 7 kg, is gained during the second trimester. In the third trimester, weight gain is about 4 to 5 kg. For the average healthy woman, the total weight gain ranges from 11 to 16 kg. Women who are underweight need to gain a little more weight while overweight women, a little less.

Distribution of Weight Gain in Pregnancy

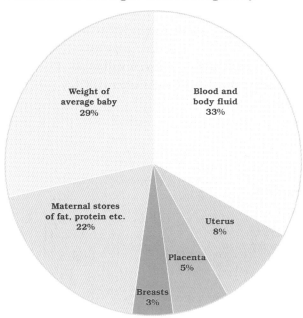

Gaining Too Little Weight

Women who do not gain enough weight during pregnancy have an increased risk of delivering small babies (birth weight of less than 2.5 kg). Smaller babies tend to have health problems such as asthma and respiratory tract infections (cough and cold). They are at greater risk of having cerebral palsy (a nervous system disorder causing difficulty in talking and walking) and their intelligence quotient (IQ) may be impaired.

Gaining Too Much Weight

Gaining too much weight in pregnancy may increase the risk of developing hypertension and gestational diabetes. The unborn baby tends to be big and this increases the risk of having a caesarean-section. Overweight babies may also become obese and diabetic later in life.

While most women tend to indulge in their favourite food during pregnancy, it is advisable to control your weight gain by eating appropriate quantities and a well-balanced diet. Not only will this make the pregnancy and birth less risky for you and your baby, it will make it easier for you to shed the extra weight after delivery.

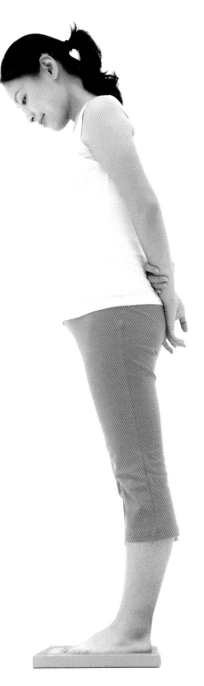

General Guidelines for Pregnancy Weight Gain

Pre-pregnancy Weight	Recommended Weight Gain
Underweight (BMI less than 18.5)	13 to 18 kg
Normal weight (BMI 18.5 to 24.9)	11 to 16 kg
Overweight (BMI 25 to 29.9)	7 to 11 kg
Obese (BMI 30 or greater)	5 to 9 kg

Source: Institute of Medicine USA

What to Take to Hospital

It is a good idea to have your bag packed and ready to go when you are in the eighth month of your pregnancy so that you will not be rushing around in a panic when you begin to have the first signs of labour.

For Yourself

* Letter of admission.

* Toothbrush and toothpaste.

* Comb or hair brush and other hair care products that you normally use.

* Moisturiser and lip balm: To keep your skin and lips moisturised as you will be staying in a fully air-conditioned environment for two to three days before you are discharged.

* Make-up: To freshen yourself up when relatives and friends come visiting after your baby is born.

* Slippers: For walking around in the room and down the corridor.

* Socks: To keep your feet warm.

* Underwear: Pack a few pairs of your old undies which you can wear and throw away if they get too soiled should your maternity napkins leak.

* Nursing bras and nursing pads.

* Maternity napkins.

* Going home outfit: Do not expect your body to shrink back to your pre-pregnancy size immediately after delivery. Make sure that the outfit you pick out is something that you can get into. If you have a caesarean-section, it will be more comfortable if you wear something loose around your waist.

* Relaxation materials: Pack a book or a few magazines and music CDs.

For Your Baby

* Baby blanket: To swaddle your baby when leaving the hospital.

* Outfit for going home.

* A pair of socks or booties.

* Newborn diapers, although most hospitals will provide you with sufficient diapers for a few days.

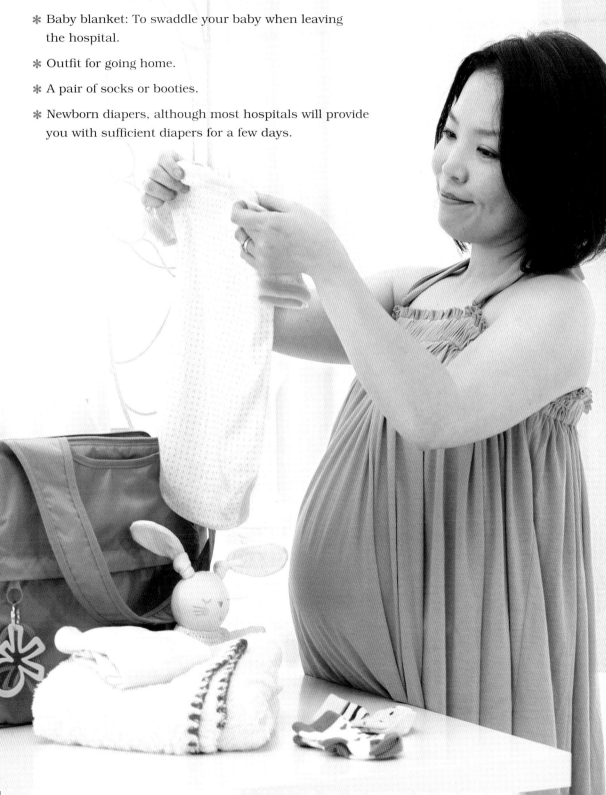

Normal Labour

One of the top concerns of pregnant women is how they will know that they are in labour, especially if it is their first pregnancy. Some women say "you just know" but here are some sure signs you can look out for to determine if you are in labour and that your baby is on the way!

Signs of Labour

Labour may begin in a number of ways. You may notice a sudden discharge of a blood-stained mucus plug, also known as "show", indicating that the cervix is beginning to dilate. Alternatively, you may start labour by having regular, frequent contractions which become progressively painful. Others may experience a sudden uncontrollable gush of water that will wet their underwear.

There are three stages of labour. The first stage is the longest, during which the cervix dilates to 10 cm. The second stage is when the head of the baby has descended deep into the pelvis to cause a "bearing down" sensation. The third stage begins after the baby is born and ends when the placenta is delivered.

First Stage

The first stage of labour starts with regular contractions and/or other signs of labour. It can be divided into the latent (quiet) and active phases.

Latent Phase

The contractions are not particularly painful and occur at 5- to 10-minute intervals. The contractions will soon become stronger with shorter intervals although your cervix is still dilating slowly.

Call your doctor and inform him of your contractions. Once your doctor confirms that you are in labour, make your way to the hospital. Your spouse will be asked to assist with the admission paperwork and you will be prepared for labour in the delivery suite. Your spouse will then get ready to join you in the delivery suite.

Active Phase

The active phase starts with more rapid dilation, normally 0.5 cm to 1 cm per hour. Once labour has begun, you will be examined vaginally at regular intervals to see how much the cervix has dilated and to assess how labour is progressing. Your baby will be monitored by a foetal heartbeat monitor. Two belts are strapped around your abdomen to record the baby's heart rate and the uterine contractions.

A pictorial record of labour, which is known as a partogram, is used once labour is established. The partogram includes a 4-hour action line recommended by the World Health Organization (WHO). This means that if the labour does not progress as predicted after four hours, action will be taken, such as breaking the water bag artificially or using labour stimulating drugs, to speed up the labour.

Second Stage

The second stage of labour starts when the cervix is fully dilated and ends with the birth of the baby.

∗ Your contractions are stronger, occurring at 2- to 5-minute intervals and last 60 to 90 seconds each time.

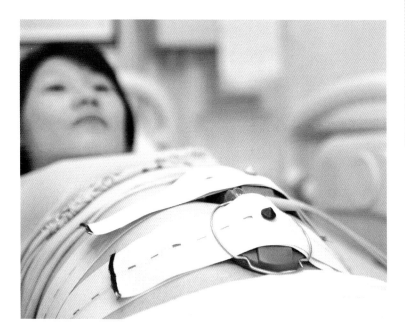

✳ The head of your baby will descend deeply into the pelvis and will rotate anteriorly so that the back of the head is behind your pubic bone.

✳ With each contraction, your baby is pushed further into the pelvis. Your baby's head will emerge first, followed by his shoulders and the rest of his body. Your baby is born!

After your baby is examined, measured and weighed, he will be placed on your chest. Take time to enjoy these precious moments with your spouse and your newborn.

Assisted Delivery

Sometimes, the second stage of labour may become prolonged and difficult. At this stage, your doctor may recommend assisted delivery in the form of forceps or ventouse for the following reasons.

• Your baby is showing signs of distress.

• You are tired and cannot push any more.

• Your baby is not making any progress through your pelvis.

• You have a medical reason why you should not push for too long, such as heart disease or previous caesarean-section.

In forceps delivery, the forceps are placed on both sides of your baby's head. At your next contraction, as you push, your doctor pulls to help your baby along.

With ventouse, a suction cap is positioned on your baby's head and a vacuum is created in the cup. Controlled traction is applied, synchronised with your contractions and pushing.

There may be pressure marks or some bruising on the baby's head from the use of the instruments for assisted delivery. But they will go away and should not cause any permanent or serious harm to your baby.

Third Stage

The third stage of labour starts with the birth of the baby and ends with the delivery of the placenta, umbilical cord and membranes from the uterus.

The placenta will usually expel on its own or it can be delivered by controlled cord traction. At the time when your baby is born, you will be given an injection of oxytocin and/or ergometrine to reduce the risk of excessive bleeding from the uterus. Choosing to wait for the spontaneous expulsion of the placenta is safe, provided you do not have excessive bleeding. It may take up to 45 minutes for the placenta to expel by itself.

If you wish to store the stem cells from baby's cord blood, your obstetrician will clamp the cord after the baby's birth and draw the blood from the placental end of the umbilical cord.

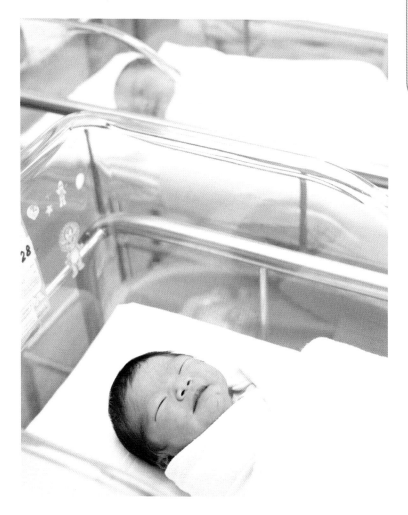

ALTERNATIVE METHODS OF BIRTHING

Besides the traditional birthing methods which involve your doctor and pain relief, some women may choose alternative birth methods such as water, hypnosis, acupressure and acupuncture, although not all methods may be available where you are.

Water Birthing

One of the more popular alternative methods of birthing today is water birthing. It is the process of giving birth in a tub of warm water. Some women choose to labour in the water and get out of the tub for delivery. Other women decide to stay in the water for the delivery as well. The theory behind water birthing is that lying in warm water can help the mother relax and cope with labour pains. The water also emulates the environment of the womb.

Many hospitals in Singapore provide hydrotherapy during labour but do not do water delivery. Check with your doctor and the hospital if you are hoping to have a water birth.

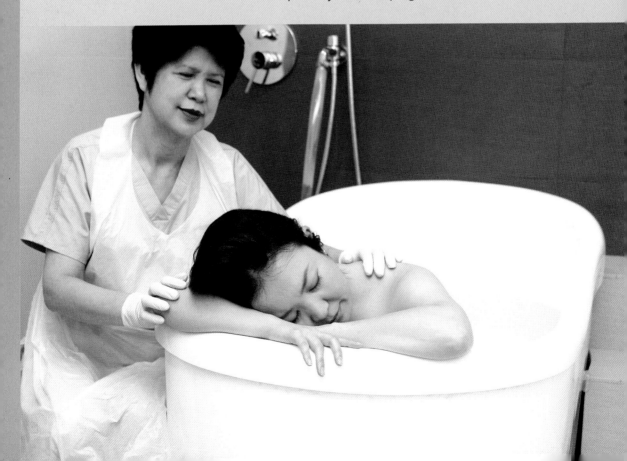

CORD BLOOD BANKING

The blood that remains in the placenta and umbilical cord after birth is referred to as cord blood. Cord blood banking is the collection and storage of this cord blood.

Stem cells in the cord blood are immature cells that can multiply and mature into other types of cells in the body, essentially replacing or treating diseased organs. Stem cells have been used to treat blood diseases and cancers since the late 1960s. This procedure was known as a bone marrow transplant then, and involved using blood stem cells from a normal donor to replace the diseased marrow in the patient.

Such treatments are now known as Stem Cell Transplants (SCT), where blood stem cells from the bone marrow, peripheral blood or cord blood are used.

How Cord Blood May Help

There is only one opportunity to bank a newborn's cord blood, and this is at birth. The cord blood collection process is painless and harmless to the baby and mother but the decision must be made before the birth of the baby.

Should there be a need for a bone marrow transplant in your family in the future, you may have a problem finding a match. By banking your newborn's stem cells, the odds of finding a suitable match for the baby or another family member improve.

Future medical advances might allow stem cells to treat even more diseases and be used in more transplant cases than being used currently.

For more information on cord blood banking, visit the Singapore Cord Blood Bank website (www.scbb.com.sg).

Pain Relief during Labour

It is a personal choice whether or not you want any form of pain relief during delivery. If you feel that you may need some form of pain relief, find out as much as you can about the different types of pain relief available to you, then make an informed choice about which one to go for.

Alternative Methods of Pain Relief

There are some women who choose not to use drugs and prefer alternative methods of pain relief such as acupuncture, aromatherapy, homeopathy, hypnosis and reflexology. Although these methods may help you relax during labour, most of these techniques do not provide very effective pain relief.

Epidural Anaesthesia

Epidural anaesthesia is the most popular means of pain relief during labour. It enables you to be fully involved in the birth of your baby without being distracted and exhausted by the pain and discomfort.

Some women, however, may not be suitable for an epidural due to medical conditions such as spinal problems or surgery, bleeding disorders and certain complications of pregnancy.

How It Works

A special epidural needle is inserted into the lower part of the back, then pushed into the space that contains the nerves before they enter the spinal cord. With the epidural needle in place, a fine plastic tube is passed through the needle, which is then withdrawn. The plastic tube is taped in place so that an anaesthetic drug can be infused continuously through it till delivery without further injections. This numbs the nerves carrying the pain sensation from the womb and birth canal.

Initially, there may be a tingling sensation or warmth in the legs which may gradually become numb and weak. The onset of pain relief starts 10 to 20 minutes from the time the anaesthetic drug is injected into the epidural catheter.

The blood pressure of the mother and the baby's heartbeat are carefully and continuously monitored. An intravenous drip is set up to prevent a sudden fall in blood pressure.

The pain relief will last until the baby is delivered. During the second stage of labour, you may feel the pressure of the baby's head descending through the birth canal. Assisted delivery (forceps or ventouse, page 58) is common as the mother often loses the sensation to push.

After the delivery, the catheter is removed. The effects of the anaesthesia usually wear off within one to two hours. After the medicine wears off, you may have an uncomfortable burning sensation around the birth canal which will stop after a while.

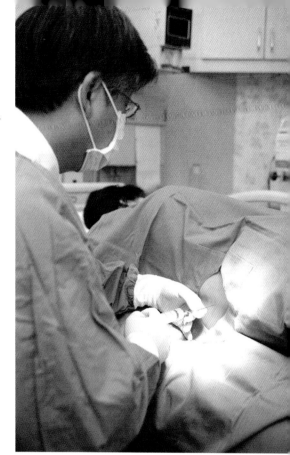

Advantages

It eliminates most of the discomfort of labour and delivery without causing giddiness or sleepiness as with the inhalation of laughing gas (nitrous oxide) or pain-killer injection (pethidine). Most women feel that they are able to participate in the labour process and are not too exhausted to bond with their baby. If an immediate caesarean-section is required, it can be performed with the epidural anaesthesia.

Risks

No anaesthetic is without risk but most patients do not suffer any serious complications. The complications are not common and can be treated immediately with careful monitoring.

* Fall in blood pressure. This is often prevented by administering an intravenous drip.

* Shivering. This is a common side effect but it is not serious.

* Itching and pain over the site of injection.

* Occasionally, the epidural needle may accidentally puncture a hole in the sac containing the spinal fluid, in which case the mother will experience a severe headache for a few days after the procedure. By using a blood patch performed by the anaesthetist, the headache will disappear quickly.

* As the nerve supply of the bladder is also anaesthetised, the patient may not be able to urinate and catheterisation may be required. Urinary catheterisation, however, increases the risk of urinary infection.

* Infection following an epidural is extremely rare and if treated early with antibiotics, recovery is usually complete and without complications.

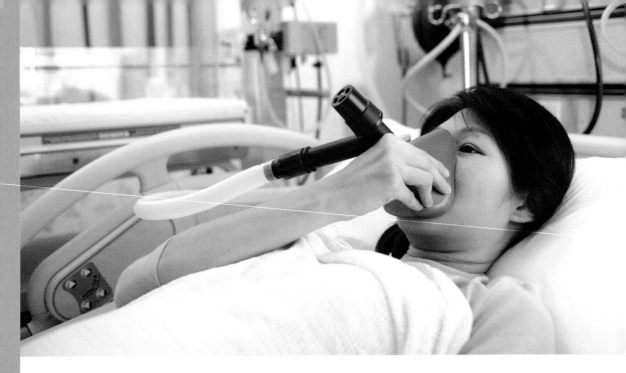

Entonox

This is a mixture of oxygen and nitrous oxide. It is used towards the end of the first stage and in the second stage of labour.

How It Works
You breathe in the gas through a face mask or mouthpiece. You take a breath of the gas just as a contraction begins.

Advantages
This form of pain relief is simple and safe and can be self-administered once the machine has been set up for you. The gas takes just 15 to 20 seconds to work and is most effective if taken in slow, deep breaths.

Risks
There are no harmful side effects on you or your baby although you may experience nausea, dizziness and disorientation. Your mouth may also feel dry as the gas is administered orally.

Pain Killers

Another form of pain relief is the intramuscular injection of pain killers such as pethidine or morphine.

How It Works

The drug is injected directly into your thigh or buttocks.
It takes about 20 minutes to become effective and will last
between two and four hours.

Advantages

These injections will help you to relax and hence lessen
the pain.

Risks

The side effects include nausea and difficulty in pushing
during the second stage of labour. If the injections are given
too close to the time of delivery, the drug may cross the
placenta and affect your baby's breathing. If this happens,
an antidote will be given to your baby. The drug can cause
drowsiness in you and your baby and, as a result, delay the
establishment of breastfeeding.

Transcutaneous Electrical Nerve Stimulation (TENS)

TENS is an alternative pain relief method that does not involve
the use of drugs. It is used during the first stage of labour.

How It Works

Electrode pads are taped on your back and connected by wires
to a small battery-powered stimulator. A low voltage electric
current is passed across these pads to stimulate your body to
produce natural pain-relieving hormones called endorphins.
It also reduces the number of pain signals that are sent to the
brain by the spinal cord. It takes about 30 minutes before any
effect is felt.

Advantages

It is non-invasive and easy to use. When you start to feel the
effects of labour, your spouse can help you put the pads on.

Risks

There are no known side effects on you or your baby but
TENS may only help during the early stage of labour as it
ceases to be effective when contractions get longer, stronger
and more frequent.

Caesarean-section

Caesarean-section is a surgical procedure to deliver the baby through an incision in the mother's abdomen. It may be planned if the mother has medical problems like heart disease or pregnancy complications such as if the baby is in an abnormal position, making vaginal delivery difficult or dangerous. Sometimes, it may be an emergency caesarean-section that is decided in the midst of labour for the safety of the mother or baby, or both.

When a Caesarean-section Is Necessary

* Labour is not progressing well. The cervix is not opening enough despite strong contractions over several hours or the baby's head may be too big to pass through the birth canal.

* Foetal distress. The baby is not getting enough oxygen or the doctor is concerned about changes in the baby's heartbeat.

* Baby is in an abnormal position. The baby is in an abnormal position inside the womb, such as the breech position, which can cause complications if delivery continues through the vagina.

* Multiple births. If the mother is carrying multiple babies, it is common for one or more of the babies to be in an abnormal position.

* Problem with placenta. If the placenta detaches from the uterus before labour begins and blocks the opening of the cervix.

* Problem with the umbilical cord. A caesarean-section may be recommended if a loop of umbilical cord slips through the cervix ahead of the baby or if the cord is compressed by the uterus during contractions.

* Mother's medical condition. If the mother has a medical condition such as diabetes or heart disease, the doctor may induce labour early to reduce the risk of pregnancy-related complications. If the induction is not successful, she may need a caesarean-section.

＊ Previous caesarean-section. Depending on the type of incision and other factors, the mother may be able to attempt a vaginal delivery after a previous caesarean section. In some cases, however, the doctor may recommend a repeat caesarean-section.

A caesarean-section can be carried out using epidural anaesthesia, although, in an emergency, general anaesthesia may be required. Recovery from a caesarean-section takes longer than recovery from a vaginal birth. As with any major surgery, it carries a higher risk of complications to the mother and baby.

Care after a Caesarean-section

In Hospital

Following your caesarean-section, you need to try to get as much rest as you can to avoid pulling on the stitches. However, you should try to move your legs while in bed and get up to use the bathroom within the first 24 hours after the surgery. This will help prevent blood clots and speed up the healing. The sutures will be removed after a week or so. Before that, your doctor will show you how to clean the wound with antiseptic solution and cover it with protective dressing to prevent infection.

You will be given medication for pain relief after surgery. Check with your doctor if you can breastfeed while on the medication. The catheter that is inserted during surgery will be removed after 12 hours or earlier. Drink plenty of water to prevent getting a UTI. If you feel up to it, you can take a short stroll outside your room. Move slowly as you may experience some dizziness.

At Home

Try not to do too much when you first get home. You will not be able to go up and down stairs or lift your baby from the cot until the wound feels less sore. In the meantime, continue to drink plenty of fluid and eat a balanced diet to restore your energy levels and prevent constipation. Avoid sexual intercourse for about six weeks as the abdominal wound and lining of the uterus need time to heal.

Post-delivery Care

Giving birth is both exhausting and emotional. While your attention is now focussed on your baby, you also need to take care of yourself. Try not to have unrealistic expectations of yourself as a parent. There will be days when you will not have the time to do everything and days when you feel you cannot cope. Take it easy and everything will be a whole lot smoother.

Physical Changes

In the first few weeks after giving birth, you may experience some physical changes as your body begins to recover.

Vaginal Soreness

If you had an episiotomy or vaginal tear during delivery, the wound may hurt for a few weeks. If sitting is uncomfortable, doughnut-shaped air rings are available from pharmacies. Sitting on the ring will help ease the pressure. You can also help promote healing by:

* Keeping the wound clean.

* Using an ice pack to soothe the wound.

* Cleaning your vulva with warm water after urinating.

See your doctor immediately if the wound becomes hot, swollen and painful or produces a pus-like discharge.

Vaginal Discharge

You will have a vaginal discharge, known as lochia, for up to six weeks after delivery. The discharge is a bright red, heavy flow of blood for the first few days. It will gradually taper off, changing from pink or brown to yellow or white. Do not be alarmed if you occasionally pass blood clots. See your doctor if the lochia becomes too heavy with large clots or has a foul smell, or if you are running a fever of 38°C or higher.

Contractions

You may continue to have contractions, called after-pains, for the first few days after delivery. These contractions are most noticeable when breastfeeding.

Urination Problems

As a result of pregnancy and vaginal delivery, the muscles that support your bladder and keep the urethra closed can be overstretched, causing you to lose control of your bladder, particularly when you cough, laugh or sneeze. Daily pelvic floor exercises will help with this problem.

Swelling or bruising of the tissues surrounding the bladder and urethra may also lead to difficulty urinating but this usually resolves on its own. Contact your doctor if you experience pain when urinating, incomplete emptying and/or a frequent urge to urinate.

Haemorrhoids

Some women may experience haemorrhoids or swollen veins in the anus or lower rectum after childbirth. To ease the discomfort, soak the affected areas with warm salted water. Your doctor may recommend a topical haemorrhoid medication as well.

To prevent constipation and straining, which contribute to haemorrhoids, eat food high in fibre, including fruit, vegetables and wholegrains, and drink plenty of water. If your stools are still hard, your doctor may recommend a stool softener or fibre laxative.

Sore Breasts and Leakage of Breast Milk

Your breasts may become heavy, swollen and tender when your milk comes in. This is known as engorgement. To ease the discomfort, nurse your baby frequently or use a breast pump to express the milk. You may also want to apply ice packs or hot towels to your breasts.

Milk leaking from the breasts is also a common problem for new mothers. You cannot do anything to stop the leaking but nursing pads worn inside your bra can help keep your top dry. Change pads after each feed and whenever they get wet.

Hair Loss and Skin Changes

During pregnancy, increased hormone levels put normal hair loss on hold. After delivery, the reverse happens and you will shed the excess hair all at once. This is a natural process and your hair growth will go back to normal within six months.

Do not expect your stretch marks to go away immediately. They will gradually fade from reddish purple to silver or white.

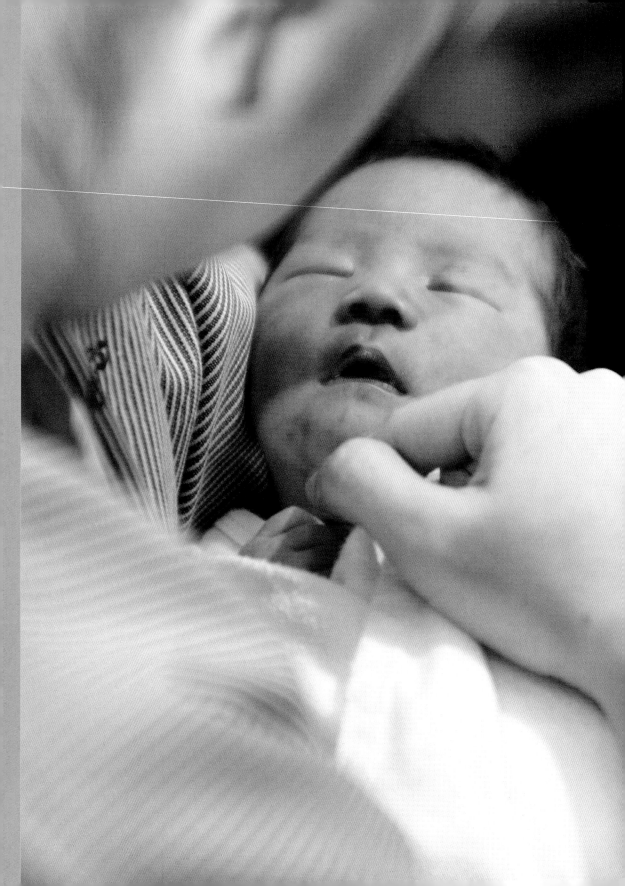

Emotional Changes

Changes in your hormone levels may make you feel tearful, irritable, depressed and tired. Between three and five days after giving birth, some women may also feel particularly low and emotional. This is referred to as the baby blues. Try to rest as much as you can, eat healthily and accept offers of help. However, if you are still feeling low or depressed after a few weeks, speak to your doctor about it.

Rest

Looking after a newborn baby is demanding. Your body is also recovering from the rigours of pregnancy and childbirth; and if you are feeding through the night, you may become exhausted. It is essential that you rest. It may be tempting to use the time when your baby sleeps during the day to catch up with chores but it is important for your well-being that you get enough sleep and rest. Leave the chores for another day or get your family or friends to help you with them.

Your Weight and Shape

Your body has undergone enormous changes during the length of your pregnancy and it is going to take as long to get your body back into shape. Soon after birth, your tummy will still be larger than it was before you became pregnant. Eating healthily will help you get on track to regain your pre-pregnancy weight and shape.

Healthy Diet

It is very important to maintain a healthy diet. Not only do you need the energy to look after your baby, a healthy diet will provide a good source of nutrients if you are breastfeeding.

Exercise

Check with your doctor when you can start exercising and try to fit exercising into your daily routine. Not only is it relaxing, it will help your body recover and help you keep fit. Walking, swimming and post-natal exercise classes are some options you may want to consider. They will help to improve your shape and strengthen your muscles.

The Postpartum Checkup

A postpartum checkup is typically scheduled six weeks after delivery. Your doctor will check your vagina, cervix and uterus to make sure that you are healing well. He will also examine your breasts and check your weight and blood pressure. Take this opportunity to talk to your doctor about exercise, birth control, breastfeeding and how you are adjusting to life with your newborn.

Preparing Baby's Room

One of the most exciting parts of preparing for the arrival of a new baby is setting up baby's room. Here is a guide to help you make your baby's room safe, functional and special.

Decorating Baby's Room

Your baby will not be able to appreciate the effort you put into decorating his room, but doing it up means you will be able to enjoy the comfort when you spend time feeding, changing and putting him to bed in his room.

* Any colour scheme will work, but it is better to go for light colours to make the room look brighter and more cheerful.

* Accessorise the room with brightly coloured curtains and bedding to make it more interesting and fun for you and your baby.

* Keep the furnishing simple so it is functional but easy to clean.

Checklist for Baby's Room

* Baby cot.

* Chest of drawers and/or cupboard for baby clothes and toiletries.

* Changing table or changing pad. It is not necessary to have a changing table as this may take up too much space. With a changing pad, you can change your baby anywhere in the home, on the floor or on the bed, whichever is more convenient.

* Comfortable chair. You may want to get a comfortable chair to sit on while feeding your baby. Or you may want to get a rocking chair where you can sit and rock your baby to sleep.

* Basket or box for toys.

* Small table lamp or night light for when you need to change or feed your baby in the room in the middle of the night.

Safety Concerns

Safety is an important consideration when doing up baby's room.

- Make sure that the furniture is sturdy and will not tip over when your baby becomes mobile and pulls on them.
- Choose furniture with rounded corners to eliminate the possibility of your baby hurting himself when he starts crawling or walking.
- Lights and fans should preferably be mounted on the wall or ceiling so there are no loose cables that your baby can pull or tug on.

* Baby monitor. Although this is not a necessity, depending on the layout of your home, it might help you monitor your baby when you are in your own room or elsewhere in the home.

A Baby Cot

You can expect your baby to sleep in the cot until he is about 18 months old or when he starts trying to climb out of it. Here are some things to look out for when buying a cot for your baby.

- The base of the cot is adjustable so you do not have to bend down too far to pick your baby up in the early months. When your baby grows older, the mattress can be lowered.

- One or both sides of the cot can be lowered for you to put down and pick up your baby easily.

- The slats are no more than 6 cm apart so that your baby's head does not go through them.

- The side rails are protected with a plastic covering for when your baby starts teething. Check that the plastic covering is tightly secured and unbroken.

- No protruding or rough edges.

- Lockable swivel castors to make it easier to move the cot around. Remember to lock the wheels when your baby is in the cot.

- The mattress fits snugly into the cot so your baby will not get his arms, legs or head caught in between the sides.

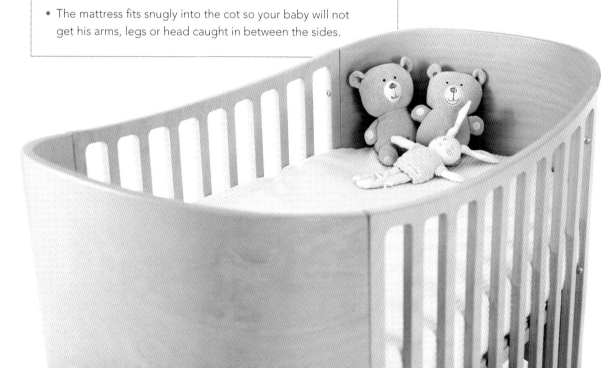

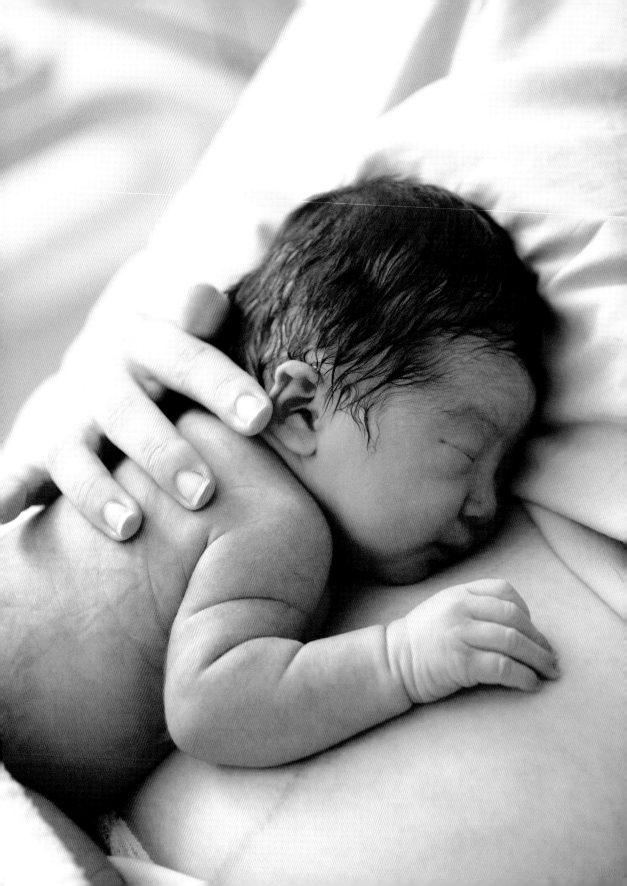

Your
Newborn

The big moment is here—the birth of your baby!
Everything goes by in a blur amid your excitement
and the flurry of activities in the delivery room.
And before you know it, you are cradling your
little bundle of joy in your arms! This chapter tells you
what happens in the delivery room, what to expect
of your newborn and the routine examination and
screening tests for your baby soon after his birth.

Contributors:

Sr Kang Phaik Gaik
Dr Yvonne Ng

| Pregnancy | 0 to 1 month | 2 to 11 months | 12 months to 3 years | 3 to 6 years |

Straight after your baby is born, he will be checked by the medical staff to ensure that all is well. He will then be handed to you to be held for the first time.

The neonatologist will physically examine your newborn usually within 24 hours after birth. This is a routine check to make sure that your baby has made the transition to life outside the womb without difficulty and to check for major congenital abnormalities.

The doctor will also listen to your baby's heart sounds and check his hips, eyes and genitalia to make sure that all is well. Talk to the neonatologist if you notice anything unusual about your baby's physical appearance.

Routine Tests

Apgar Score

The Apgar score is an assessment of a newborn based on five signs—breathing, heart rate, colour, muscle tone and reflexes. Every sign is given a score of 0, 1 or 2. Total scores at 1 minute and 5 minutes after birth are usually recorded to document the newborn's transition after birth and response to resuscitation if the latter is necessary. Most babies born without any need for resuscitation, score about 9 at 5 minutes of life. The full score of 10 is unusual because most babies still have slightly blue hands and feet due to the cold environment outside the womb.

Apgar scores below 7 indicate a baby who is "depressed". If the Apgar score continues to be low, a neonatologist will be on hand to step up resuscitation efforts. The Apgar score is generally not used to predict long-term neurological development of the baby as most "depressed" newborns go on to develop normally.

G6PD and Low Thyroid Hormone Levels

From the cord blood, tests are carried out for G6PD (page 83) and low thyroid hormone levels. One in 4,000 babies has very low thyroid hormone levels due to absent thyroid gland tissue or problems with thyroid hormone production. When detected early, hormone replacement (thyroxine) can be started immediately and continued throughout life to maintain normal growth and development of the child.

Hearing

All newborns undergo the Universal Newborn Hearing Screening Programme for early detection of severe and moderate hearing loss.

If your baby passes the hearing screening test, it means that your baby's hearing function is normal at the time of testing.

If your baby does not pass this screening test, further testing is needed. Early detection of hearing problems and appropriate intervention will result in good speech and development, even for children with hearing abnormalities.

Inborn Errors of Metabolism (IEM)

The latest newborn screening test is the Inborn Errors of Metabolism (IEM), which screens for about 25 disorders of body chemistry. Metabolic disorders are rare. The estimated incidence in Singapore is about one in 3,000 to 4,000 babies. However, individuals affected by an IEM disorder will have difficulty processing nutrients normally and may develop serious medical problems like mental and physical disabilities and even death.

Most babies with IEM disorders are healthy at birth. It will be several days or months before they become sick. Early detection and treatment with special diet and medication are important to prevent serious medical harm.

Other Routine Procedures

Parents will be asked for written consent to give their newborn the BCG and hepatitis B vaccinations after birth. The BCG is to protect against severe tuberculosis infection while the hepatitis B vaccination is the first dose in a series of three (at birth, 1 month and 6 months) to provide hepatitis B immunity. When you are discharged from hospital, you will be given a health booklet to record your baby's immunisations and visits to the doctor for growth and developmental checks.

Although the skin of a baby is soft and supple, it is not necessarily blemish-free. Babies often have rashes and blemishes which, in most cases, will go away without treatment.

Skin

The full-term newborn will be covered in vernix, a sticky white substance that provides a natural moisture barrier. After his bath, he will look more pink. Some babies may have dry skin with superficial peeling or cracks, especially if they are born past 42 weeks.

Newborn Acne

Babies often develop a harmless case of acne on their forehead, chin and cheeks. This common skin condition is called acne neonatorum. It is believed to be due to stimulation of the sebaceous glands by maternal hormones and usually resolves by the baby's fourth month without scarring. Treatment is not needed unless the rash is severe or shows no sign of getting better.

Milia

Milia or milk spots are tiny white lumps found on the face. They are caused by the retention of old skin cells and oily substances within the hair follicles. Leave them alone. They should clear up within your baby's first month of life.

Heat Rash

Some babies are prone to getting heat rash or prickly heat during hot weather. The rash usually starts around the neck. If it is bad, it can spread down to the chest and back and up around the ears and face.

Most forms of heat rash do not require any treatment. Just wipe the skin with cool water and pat dry. You can also dust the affected areas with baby powder that contains corn flour as this will help absorb excess moisture. Prevent your baby from getting heat rash by dressing him lightly and keeping him cool.

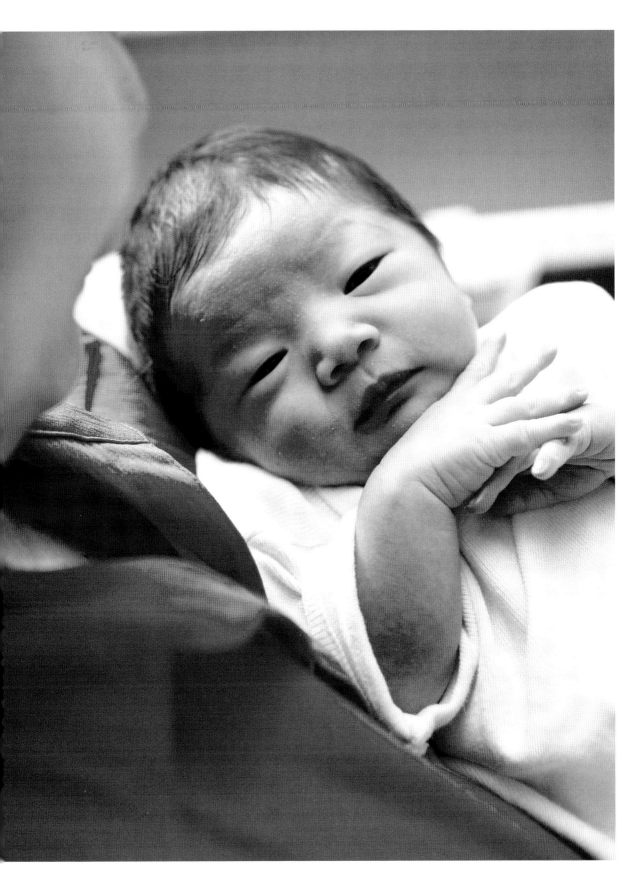

Erythema Toxicum

This is a rash that appears as small pus-filled spots on the baby's trunk and limbs, usually during the first few days after birth. If your baby is otherwise well and not bothered by the rash, leave it alone and it will disappear by the first month of life. But if your baby is unwell with symptoms such as fever and irritability and is not feeding well, take him to the doctor as the rash may be due to a bacterial, viral or fungal infection that will require prompt treatment.

Scalp

There is likely to be some swelling in the scalp due to the prolonged labour and the squeeze through the birth canal, but this will resolve within a few days.

You may also notice a soft swelling usually located on one side of your baby's scalp. This is due to a collection of blood over the skull bone layer following prolonged labour or assisted vacuum or forceps delivery. This is known as cephalhaematoma. There is no need to massage this swelling to try and reduce it. Depending on its size, it will resolve on its own after a few weeks. It does not affect your baby's head or brain growth but he may become a little jaundiced when the blood is broken down and reabsorbed into his body.

Cradle Cap

Cradle cap refers to the condition where the baby's scalp is covered with yellow greasy scales. The lesions can also affect the face, neck and ears. The condition tends to be self-limiting and resolves spontaneously within a few weeks or months. Most of the time, no treatment is required. If desired, the scales can be softened with olive oil and then removed with a soft brush prior to washing the scalp. Special shampoos are also available for treating persistent or severe cradle cap.

Epstein Pearls

Epstein pearls are tiny white or yellow lumps that appear along the gums or hard palate inside the baby's mouth. They will disappear of their own accord after about a month.

THE LATE PRETERM BABY

About 7 percent of babies in Singapore are born prematurely. The majority of them are born three to five weeks before their due date. These babies are referred to as "late preterm" babies.

Although late preterm babies may be similar in size and weight as full-term babies, they are considered "at risk" because they are physiologically and metabolically less mature. They will need to be closely monitored in hospital for at least 48 hours after birth.

Depending on the baby's condition, the neonatologist will decide whether he needs to be observed in the normal nursery, special care nursery or neonatal intensive care unit. Many neonatology departments have standard guidelines for admitting babies born between 34 and 35 weeks into the special care nursery.

Breathing and Feeding Difficulties

Some late preterm babies may have breathing difficulties soon after birth and require oxygen or breathing assistance. This could be due to insufficient lung maturity or delay in normal lung fluid re-absorption.

As the baby may also have feeding difficulties, his blood sugars will be monitored regularly for the first day of life, especially if he has a low birth weight and needs intravenous fluid infusions. He may also need additional warmth to maintain normal body temperature in the first few days.

Discharge from Hospital

A late preterm baby will be allowed to be discharged from hospital when his vital signs are stable—normal breathing and heart rate with normal body temperature in an open cot.

The baby will undergo the routine newborn screenings and be vaccinated before he leaves the hospital. Parents will be given specific instructions for his care upon discharge. It is likely that he will have an early follow-up appointment in the hospital within one to three days to make sure that all is well.

Nutrition

The goal of optimal nutrition for premature babies is to mimic the supply of nutrition in the womb. The preferred source of nutrition is breast milk as it is well tolerated and delivers many important nutritive factors that help support the immunity of the little infant. Due to the rapid growth that needs to take place to achieve the growth he would otherwise have undergone in the womb, breast milk needs to be fortified with specialised add-on nutritive powder called human milk fortifier.

Preterm infants achieve better length, weight, head circumference measures as well as improved bone density with optimised nutrition support of a human milk fortifier than those fed breast milk alone. If breast milk is unavailable, special formulas are needed to achieve optimal nutrition for preterm infants.

Working closely with the health care team in the hospital, a mother can deliver breast milk to nourish her little one. After discharge, parents will be given special instructions to continue to fortify breast milk or provide a specialised post-discharge formula if breast milk is unavailable. This is so that the baby can catch up on the rate of growth of infants of the same gestational age who are born at term. Regular follow-up consultations with the care team during the first year of life is important to support optimal nutrition and achieve good physical and mental development outcomes in the long term for the preterm infant.

G6PD

G6PD deficiency is an inherited condition in which the body does not have enough of the enzyme glucose-6-phosphate dehydrogenase (G6PD), which helps red blood cells function normally.

It is passed down from mothers who are carriers of this condition. Their male babies have a 50 percent chance of being G6PD deficient or normal while their female babies have a 50 percent chance of being a G6PD deficient carrier or normal. It is a lifelong condition and children affected will have to observe their intake of food and medication to conserve what little G6PD they have in their bodies.

About 5 percent of Singaporean Chinese males and 3 percent of Singaporean Malay males are G6PD deficient. It is rare in the Indian ethnic group but found also in babies of Thai, Filipino and Burmese descent.

Babies with G6PD

In the baby who is G6PD deficient, the red cell membrane is more likely to break down and produce higher levels of jaundice, which can lead to brain damage. Therefore, babies who are G6PD deficient are monitored in the hospital nursery for at least 72 hours of life. The parents are counselled about the condition and informed about the need to avoid drugs and certain food that trigger red cell breakdown and how to monitor jaundice.

Parents will be provided with a list of drugs and food that babies with G6PD deficiency must avoid. This includes contact with mothballs, consumption of fava beans, sulpha drugs, antimalarials and some herbal preparations. Mothers who are breastfeeding their G6PD deficient baby will also need to avoid intake of these specific food and drugs.

Most people with G6PD deficiency do not have any symptoms while some may develop symptoms of anaemia when they are exposed to triggers such as certain food/or and drugs. Some children may require a transfusion. Only in rare cases will G6PD deficiency lead to chronic anaemia. With the right precautions, a child with G6PD deficiency can lead a healthy and active life.

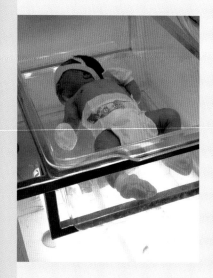

JAUNDICE IN BABIES

The liver processes bilirubin in the blood and changes it into a harmless form that is passed out of the body in faeces and urine. In newborns, the liver is immature and cannot break down the bilirubin fast enough, resulting in jaundice.

Jaundice causes the baby's skin and the white part of the eyes to appear yellow. In newborns, this yellow colour starts to appear first on the face, then chest and tummy and lastly on the legs and hands as the level of bilirubin rises.

Jaundice occurs naturally in all newborns. It starts on day three of the baby's life, reaches its peak level by day five and resolves by day seven or eight. In this normal pattern, the jaundice level is not high and does not need treatment. This is called "physiological" or normal jaundice. However, in the Singaporean Chinese ethnic group, up to 30 percent of babies will develop obvious jaundice and 15 to 20 percent may have to undergo phototherapy during the newborn period.

Other Causes of Jaundice

Breastfeeding jaundice is seen in breastfed babies in the first week, especially in those that are not nursing often enough. The baby is dehydrated with excessive weight loss and shows evidence of poor passage of meconium and reduced urine output. Early and frequent breastfeeding greatly helps to reduce this type of jaundice. The colostrum that the baby receives from breastfeeding in the first days after birth will help the baby eliminate bilirubin through the faeces.

If the baby's jaundice continues to rise after two weeks and his faeces is pale and urine dark, an urgent review is needed, as this could be due to liver disease or the blockage of bile ducts.

Excessive breakdown of red cells due to the incompatibility of the blood group of mother and child, premature birth or G6PD deficiency are some of the other causes of jaundice. In many of these cases, treatment with phototherapy is usually started during the hospital stay, and specific advice will be given to parents to monitor the child at home and return for a follow-up check where necessary.

Although complications are rare, severe infant jaundice or poorly treated jaundice can cause brain damage.

Treatment for Jaundice

If the baby's bilirubin level is high, phototherapy will be advised to treat the jaundice. This is when the baby is undressed and placed under a phototherapy unit using blue spectrum light. It usually takes 24 hours and requires the baby to stay in hospital.

He will be taken out intermittently for feeding and changing during this period. Additional blood tests will be done to find out the cause of jaundice. There is no other equally effective and safe way of treating jaundice. Medications and glucose water do not reduce bilirubin levels.

Breastfeeding and Jaundice

Unless jaundice levels are very high, breastfeeding can continue together with phototherapy. Check with the hospital if it can be arranged for you to be admitted so you can remain close to your newborn and continue breastfeeding.

The paediatrician may recommend additional fluid to supplement your breastfeeding. This is especially so if the doctor diagnosed inadequate breast milk as a contributing factor to your baby's jaundice. Do not fret but continue to breastfeed your baby and/or express your breast milk regularly eight to 12 times daily while adhering to the paediatrician's advice to supplement with additional fluid during phototherapy.

If you are separated from your newborn during the phototherapy re-admission, express your milk regularly to ensure continuity of your milk supply and to avoid breast engorgement. Let your paediatrician and nurses know that you intend to continue latching on for breastfeeding. Ask that your baby not be fed using a bottle to avoid him refusing the breast later on. Nurses are adept at feeding using a syringe or cup in hospital. The milk fed can be your expressed breast milk or formula milk.

After phototherapy is completed, your baby will be discharged from hospital. An appointment will be made for a bilirubin level check within the next few days.

You may have talked frequently to your baby while he was still in your womb and seen him on the ultrasound screen during your prenatal visits to the doctor, but the journey of getting to know your baby only really begins once you are home. You may be overwhelmed by the responsibility of caring for your newborn but your emotions are normal. Take time to adjust to being a mum and bond with your baby by cuddling and caressing him. Here are some physical changes that you may notice in your baby in his first week home.

Skin Rashes

Within the next few days, a common skin rash called erythema toxicum neonatorum may appear and your baby's skin will have splotchy red areas with yellow-white pustules in the centre. This is not a skin infection and will go away in a few days. A heat rash may also appear around your newborn's neck or body, especially during warm weather or if you cover up your baby too much.

Umbilical Stump

The umbilical stump dries up and eventually detaches by about a week after birth. Use a clean cotton bud to dry the area around the stump after a bath. There is no need to use any antiseptic lotion or powder. Expose the stump to air to help dry out the base. Keep the front of your baby's diaper folded away from the stump.

During the healing process, it is normal to see a little crust or dried blood near the stump. Consult a doctor if your baby develops a fever or if the umbilical area appears red and swollen, continues to bleed, oozes pus or produces a foul-smelling discharge.

Eye Discharge

Mild eye discharge is normal. It can be cleaned off easily with cotton wool dipped in cool boiled water. However, if the eye discharge increases or results in the swelling of the eyelids, your baby may have an eye infection. You should then take him to the doctor.

Mild eye discharge or frequent tearing of the eyes is usually due to a normal blockage in the passageway between the nose and tear gland, called the nasolacrimal duct. Excess tears will 'spill-over' as they cannot drain into the nose. The nasolacrimal duct will spontaneously open up when the baby is about 6 months old. There is no need to worry about this. Your doctor can advise you on massage techniques if the tearing persists.

Breast Enlargement

Newborn boys and girls may develop mild breast enlargement over the first few weeks due to the effects of the mother's hormones. At times, milk may drip, be visible or naturally expressed. Leave the breasts alone and the swelling will come down on its own. However, if the breast area looks red and swollen, see your doctor about it.

Vaginal Bleeding in Girls

Some baby girls may have mucous discharge from the vagina, occasionally with a tinge of blood. This occurs as the hormone oestrogen, which was passed by the mother to the baby while in the womb, begins to disappear. The discharge will last for only a few days.

THE DIAPER DECODER

Are you concerned about your baby's stool? Use this Diaper Decoder to know what is normal.

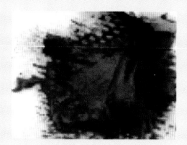

Greenish-black and Sticky

Meconium, which looks like liquorice or tar, is the first stool after birth and is perfectly normal, healthy and temporary.

What to do?

Check with your doctor if it lasts more than three days.

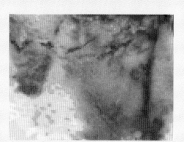

Yellow and Seedy

Breastfed baby stool is bright yellow and mild-smelling and may come with loud, even explosive, side effects. This totally normal stool is the gold standard for babies.

What to do?

Be proud.

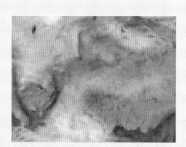

Tan and Thick

This normal, healthy stool, which looks like hummus, is the by-product of a diet that contains formula.

What to do?

You should be concerned only if the stool becomes hard or is watery.

Bowel and Bladder Movements

The table below is a general guide to your baby's pattern of urine and bowel output if you are fully breastfeeding him. Take the opportunity to change your baby's diaper in the hospital to familiarise yourself with the process and also to note your newborn's urine and bowel movements.

In the first few days, you may see a pink stain on your baby's diapers from the urine. This is due to the presence of urate crystals in the concentrated urine and is not blood.

Day of Life	Wet Diapers (per day)	Bowel Movements (per day)
First 24 hours	1	1 meconium
Day 2	2	2 meconium
Day 3	3	3 stools, colour/ consistency change
Day 4	4, light yellow	3 to 4 stools, colour/ consistency change
Day 5	5, colourless	3 to 4 yellow stools
Day 6 and beyond	6 and more, colourless	More than 4 yellow stools which may appear watery

Breastfeeding Your Baby

Breast milk is the ideal food for your baby because its nutritional composition changes throughout lactation to meet your baby's needs as he grows and develops.

Breast Milk Is Best

There is no perfect substitute for breast milk. Apart from providing your baby with the exact nourishment he needs, breast milk contains antibodies that will help your baby fight against infections and allergies.

Breastfeeding also creates a unique bond between mother and baby. Look at your baby when you breastfeed him. Smile and talk to him as he is suckling. In time, he will associate the pleasure of feeding with the sight of your face, the sound of your voice and the smell of your skin.

It is recommended that babies be fully fed on breast milk at least for the first six months of life to achieve optimal growth, development and health. After this time, your baby will need other food to meet his nutritional requirements, but breastfeeding can continue for as long as desired.

Colostrum

In the first few days of breastfeeding, colostrum is produced. It is a thick and sticky, yellowish fluid rich in antibodies to protect your baby from illness while his own immune system develops.

Transitional Milk

Transitional milk comes in three to four days after your baby is born. During this period, your baby needs to feed as often as every hour. This frequency of feeding will help to increase and establish your milk supply.

Mature Milk

After the transitional milk comes the mature milk, which is made up of two parts. At the beginning of the feed, your baby receives fore-milk to quench his thirst. As he continues to suckle from the same breast, he will receive hind milk, which is thicker with more fat to satisfy his hunger.

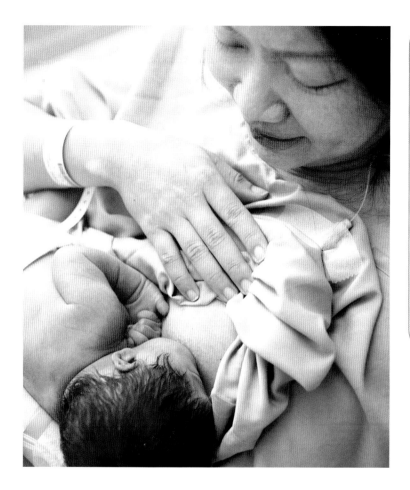

Prepare Yourself for Breastfeeding

Make the decision to breastfeed while you are pregnant to mentally prepare yourself. Get the support of your spouse and other family members. Apart from moral and emotional support, they can help out with some of the household chores so that you can get some rest between feeds.

Talk to your doctor and friends with babies about their experiences. Inform the hospital staff that you intend to breastfeed when you are admitted during labour.

As soon as your baby is born, ask the nurse to let you hold your baby directly against your chest, skin to skin, and hold him for the next hour or so. This will calm you and your baby, and normalise his temperature, heart rate and breathing. When he shows signs that he is ready to suckle, help him attach for your first breastfeed. As he suckles, your body will naturally produce more breast milk.

Breastfeeding

Newborns should not go more than four hours without feeding during the day. You should feed your baby whenever he appears hungry. Crying is a late sign of hunger. Do not wait until your baby is upset and crying from hunger before you feed him because then you have to calm him before you can feed him.

However, it does not mean that every time your baby cries, he is hungry. If he is crying only an hour after his last feed, it may be something else that is upsetting him. It may be that he just needs a cuddle or his diaper needs changing. He could also be over-stimulated, bored or too hot or too cold.

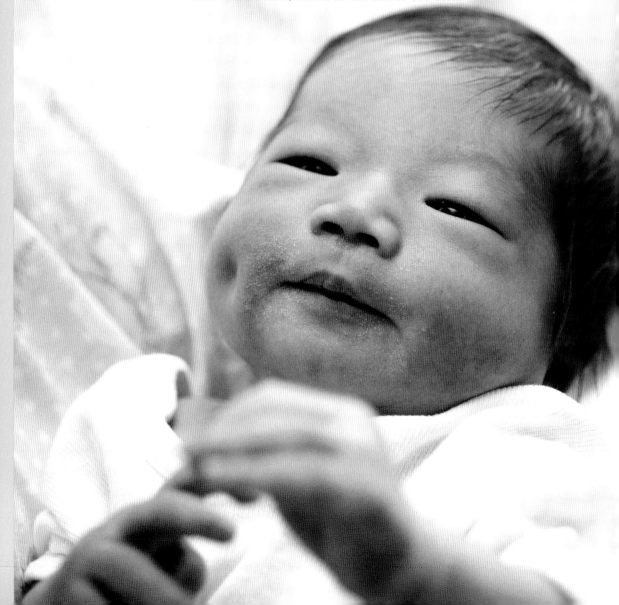

You can tell that your baby is hungry when he:

* Moves his head from side to side.

* Opens his mouth.

* Sticks out his tongue.

* Puckers his lips as if to suck.

* Nuzzles against your breast.

* Places his hands and fists to his mouth.

* Shows the rooting reflex or moves his mouth in the direction of something stroking or touching his cheek.

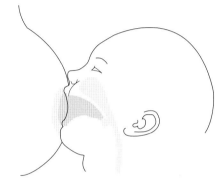

When suckling, your baby should draw both your nipple and areola into his mouth.

Latching On

Tease your baby's lips with your nipple, from his nose to his lower lip, until he opens his mouth wide. Aim your nipple at the roof of your baby's mouth and bring him towards you so that he can grasp with his mouth as much of the areola as possible into his mouth. This lets him squeeze the milk ducts under your areola.

When your baby is latched on correctly, both lips should cover nearly all of the areola with his chin resting on the lower half of your breast. Make sure that his nose is not pressed against your breast. If it is, either gently press your breast just above the areola, away from your baby's face, or bring his legs closer to you to adjust his position and free his nose. You will know that your baby is suckling well when you can see the sucking, swallowing and breathing motion.

Do not despair if the breastfeeding does not go smoothly at first. It takes a while to get it fully established. In the meantime, be patient and persevere.

Breastfeeding Positions

Find a position that is comfortable for you and your baby. It may take a few days before you discover what works best for the both of you.

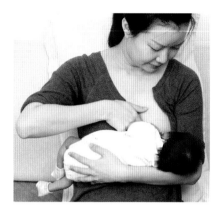

Cradle Hold

The cradle hold is the commonly used position for a good size baby and a mother with protruding nipples. Support your baby in the crook of your arm with his buttocks in your hand. Hold your baby at breast level with his face and body turned towards you.

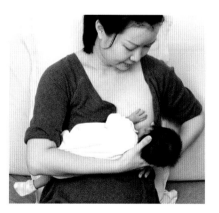

Cross Cradle Hold

This position is ideal for a small baby or a mother with short nipples. Support your baby's buttocks with your forearm and the lower part of his head, neck and back with your hand.

Football Hold

Support your back with a pillow and place another two pillows on your side. To feed your baby, hold him sideways facing you, with his torso under your armpit, and use your hand to position his head. This hold is suitable for small babies and mothers with short nipples or who had a caesarean-section.

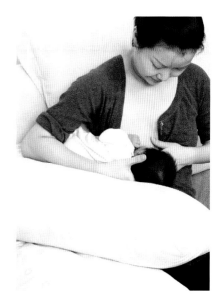

How Much Breast Milk

First-time mothers usually fret about whether their babies are getting enough breast milk. If your baby is feeding enough, he will pass clear urine regularly (six to eight times a day) and pass stools two to four times a day after the first week.

In their second or third month, some breastfed babies may not move their bowels every day and that is normal too. As long as your baby appears contented, you should not worry about him being malnourished.

Take Your Cue from Baby

Breast milk is more digestible than formula milk and therefore your baby needs to be fed more often. Your newborn should be nursing eight to 12 times per day for the first month or so.

By 1 to 2 months of age, your baby will probably suckle seven to nine times a day. As he grows older, he will suckle less frequently, and in time, develop a more reliable schedule. Some babies may suckle every one-and-a-half hours whereas others may go two or three hours between feeds.

When your baby has had enough, he will become uninterested, suckling slowly and turning away from the breast. This is the cue that you can stop feeding him.

Expressing Breast Milk

If your baby is fed solely on breast milk, expressing your milk after four to six weeks of direct latching enables another person to take over the feeding when you go back to work after your maternity leave ends. While you are still breastfeeding, offer your baby a bottle of your breast milk gradually, such as a single feed a day for one to two weeks, and slowly increase the number of bottle feeds before you go back to work.

Expressing by Hand

Most mothers choose to use a breast pump for ease and convenience, but knowing how to express by hand will ensure you can still express your milk even if your pumps do not work or if you are caught up somewhere with full breasts and do not have your baby or pump with you.

Have ready a sterilised wide-mouth container to collect the milk. Wash your hands and place your thumb and finger on the edge of the areola and press down on the milk ducts behind the areola. This should be the same spot where your baby's gums are when he is latching on. When you have emptied one breast, move on to the next breast. Your milk may spray in all directions but try to aim it as much as you can into the container.

Using a Pump

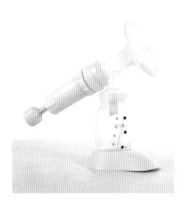

Manual and electric breast pumps are widely available today. There are many different types of pumps and the prices vary as greatly, so if you are keen to get a pump, ask around and check with your friends to see what they have found useful.

Manual breast pumps are easy to carry around and you do not need to plug them in for them to work. However, the time taken to express milk manually is longer and this may not be ideal if you are expressing at work.

Electric pumps are designed to imitate a baby's suckling action and may be a good option if you're going back to work and want to continue breastfeeding.

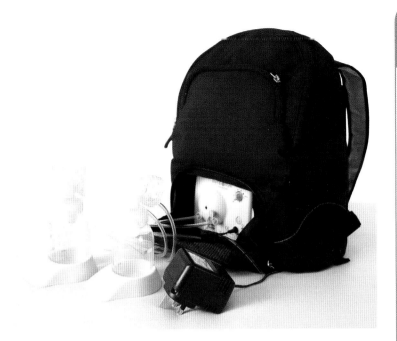

Choose a pump that best suits your needs and practise expressing your milk a few weeks before going back to work. This will enable you to get used to the process and understand how long it takes.

Storing Breast Milk

Breast milk can be kept at room temperature for up to four hours or in the refrigerator for up to 48 hours. It can be stored in the freezer for up to three months and in a deep freezer for up to six months.

Thawing Breast Milk

Thaw frozen milk in the lower compartment of your fridge for eight hours. Do not thaw milk at room temperature as it will encourage the growth of bacteria. Before feeding, bring the milk to the right temperature by placing the bottle in a bowl of warm water. Once thawed, the milk must be consumed within 24 hours. Do not refreeze it. Discard any excess milk left in the bottle after a feed.

Breastfeeding and Returning to Work

If you are planning to go back to work, you should try to breastfeed exclusively for the first four to six weeks to establish and maintain your milk supply.

After six weeks, express your milk and feed it to your baby in a bottle once a day for one to two weeks. Gradually increase the number of expressed milk feeds every week according to the number of direct feeds your baby will be missing when you are away in the office.

Continue to breastfeed your baby before and after work to maintain your milk supply. At work, set a regular schedule such as during lunch break and another one or two more times during the day to express your milk.

Store the milk in the refrigerator and take it home in a cooler box or bag with an ice pack. Transfer the milk to the refrigerator once you are home.

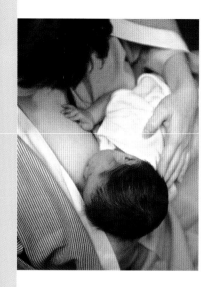

Caring for Your Breasts

It is important to care for your breasts and nipples when breastfeeding.

* After breastfeeding, rub some milk on your nipples and air-dry to soothe sensitive nipples.

* Avoid using soap on your nipples when showering as this can dry the skin and aggravate sore or cracked nipples.

* Wear a good breastfeeding bra that fits well and will support your enlarged breasts.

* When your milk supply is established, you may experience leaks of breast milk throughout the day. Nursing pads inserted into your bra will help to soak up the excess milk. Change the pads often to keep your breasts dry.

When You Are Ill

Inform your doctor that you are breastfeeding. He will prescribe medication that enables you to continue breastfeeding and provide you with the necessary advice. If you are feeling unwell and need some uninterrupted rest or sleep, you can express your milk and have someone else feed the baby.

Possible Problems

Breastfeeding should be a pleasant experience for you and your baby. However, it is not unusual to encounter some problems, especially in the beginning. Contact the lactation consultant in the hospital where you delivered your baby and she will be able to help you.

Sore Nipples

This may be due to your baby not latching on properly. Make sure that your baby has the nipple and areola well into his mouth. At the end of the feed, break the suction by gently inserting a finger into the side of his mouth. Keep your nipples as dry as possible between feeds. Be patient and persevere.

Engorgement

It is quite common that your breasts may become swollen, hard and painful on the third or fourth day. You can reduce the swelling with cold packs or chilled cabbage leaves. Gently soften the areola by expressing some milk before feeding to relieve the fullness.

Blocked Milk Duct

If you feel a painful lump in your breast, it could be due to a blocked milk duct. To clear it, press on the affected area gently and massage in circular motions and strokes towards the nipple.

You can avoid this problem by feeding often and offering your baby the affected breast first. Get him to empty your breasts at every feed. Make sure that your bra fits correctly. Avoid wearing an underwire bra or a bra that is too tight as it may press on the duct and cause it to be constricted.

Mastitis

Mastitis is an infection of the breast tissue that results in breast pain, swelling, warmth and redness of the breast. You may also have a fever with flu-like symptoms such as chills, feeling cold and body aches. See your doctor and let him know that you are breastfeeding. He may prescribe safe antibiotics to clear up the infection. In the meantime, you should continue to breastfeed.

Breast Abscess

Blocked ducts and mastitis can result in a breast abscess. It may cause you to run a fever. See your doctor who may prescribe antibiotics. If the abscess does not clear up, it may have to be drained surgically. You can continue to breastfeed using the other breast.

Breastfeeding Support Groups

Should you require peer support for breastfeeding, get in touch with local volunteer groups such as the Breastfeeding Mothers' Support Group Singapore (BMSG) and Joyful Parenting.

Formula-feeding

Breast milk offers the best in terms of nutrition for your baby and you should breastfeed for as long as possible. However, if you are unable to breastfeed, you should consult your doctor on which formula to use.

Types of Formula Milk

Most formula milk is made from a base of cow's milk. While formula milk cannot replicate breast milk, it contains a balance of nutrients, vitamins and minerals that meets your growing baby's needs.

Formula milk for babies up to 6 months old is typically labelled "Infant Formula". Infant formula is formulated to be easily digested by young babies.

"Follow On Formula" is formulated for babies after 6 months of age. Infants after the age of 6 months should start to receive supplemental foods in addition to the formula.

Preparing Formula Milk

* Wash your hands well before preparing formula for your baby.

* Fill the sterilised feeding bottle with the correct amount of boiled water and formula using the scoop provided. Level off each scoopful with a knife. Do not pack the formula into the scoop.

* Screw the cap and teat on the bottle and swirl the bottle around to dissolve the formula. Make sure the mixture is smooth and there are no lumps of formula left.

* Never add extra formula to make the milk more concentrated as this can cause your baby to fall ill or become constipated.

Tips on Bottle-feeding

* Sit comfortably and hold your baby with his head in the crook of your arm, a little higher than the rest of his body, and support his back with your forearm.

* Always give your baby freshly made formula. Test the temperature of the milk with a few drops on your wrist. It should feel comfortably warm.

* Tilt the bottle to fill the teat with milk so that your baby does not take in too much air.

* Burp him halfway through feeding and again at the end.

* After a feed, throw away any leftover milk.

* Never leave your baby with the bottle propped on a pillow. Not only is this dangerous, your baby will miss out on the cuddling that he should enjoy while he feeds.

Sterilising Feeding Equipment

As their immune systems are not fully developed, young babies are highly susceptible to infection. Any equipment you use to prepare your baby's food should be thoroughly cleaned and sterilised.

Wash your baby's milk bottle with soapy water as soon as possible after a feed. Scrub the inside of the bottle with a bottle brush and clean the teats with a teat brush to remove any traces of milk. Rinse well before sterilising.

Sterilise your baby's feeding equipment either using a steam steriliser (or a microwave steriliser, if the feeding equipment is microwave-safe) or boil it. Choose a method that is convenient for you.

BPA-free Milk Bottles

Bisphenol A (BPA) is a chemical used in the manufacture of polycarbonate plastic food and beverage containers.

There are concerns that BPA used in the plastic to make many types of milk and drink bottles could cause health problems in infants and young children.

To play it safe, you may want to use glass or look for BPA-free plastic baby bottles. And remember to change your baby's milk bottle every four to six months.

Bathing Your Baby

Bathing your newborn baby for the first time can be exciting and just a wee bit daunting, but with practise, bath time will soon become one of your favourite activities. Take the opportunity during bath time to relax, have fun and bond with your baby.

Frequency and Timing

Given our hot and humid weather, it is important to give your baby a bath at least once a day to keep him clean and fresh. Give your baby his bath before his feed if possible, as bathing him too soon after a feed may cause him to throw up.

Preparing the Bath

You can bathe your baby in any room that is warm enough and draught-free. Use a special baby bathtub with a non-slip surface and place it on a stable worktop at a height that is comfortable for you so you do not have to bend over too much.

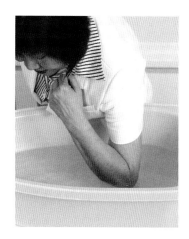

Have everything you need for the bath ready before you start. There is no need to use soap. You may want to start using baby toiletries when your baby is about 6 weeks old.

The Bath Water

Fill the bathtub first with cold water followed by hot water. Mix the water well. Test the temperature by dipping your elbow into the water. It should be comfortably warm and not too hot. Keep the water level low.

Getting Baby Ready

Place your baby on a clean bath towel on top of a protective sheet. The protective sheet will keep your worktop clean should your baby urinate or move his bowel when his diaper is removed. Gently undress him. Leave his diaper on for now and wrap him up in the towel.

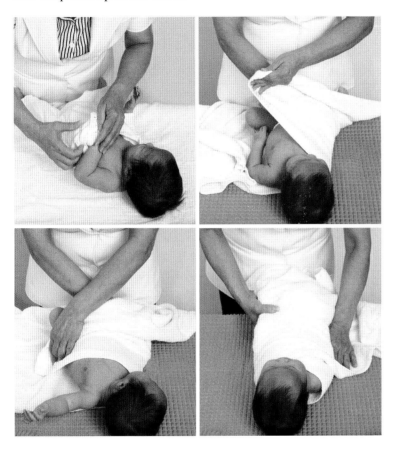

Cleaning Baby's Eyes

Make sure your hands are clean. Dip a piece of cotton wool into a bowl of cool boiled water and squeeze it dry. Clean your baby's eyes with the cotton wool starting from the inner corner of the eye and moving outwards. Use a separate piece of cotton wool for each eye.

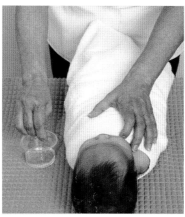 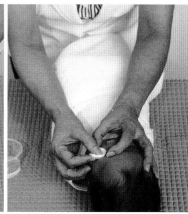

Cleaning Baby's Face and Head

Support your baby (still with the towel and diaper on) in one arm, with his head and neck in your palm. Dip a new piece of cotton wool into the water and gently squeeze it dry. Clean your baby's face from the centre outwards.

Tilt your baby's head back slightly over the tub to prevent the water from dripping down his face. Wet a piece of cotton wool and use it to gently wash his head. Washing your baby's head will help clear any cradle cap.

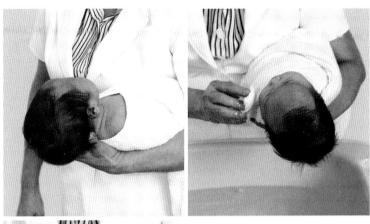

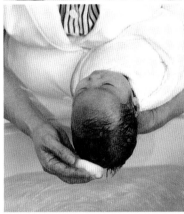

Cleaning Baby's Ears

After cleaning your baby's head, proceed to clean his ears, using a new piece of cotton wool. Clean inside his ears, then behind his ears.

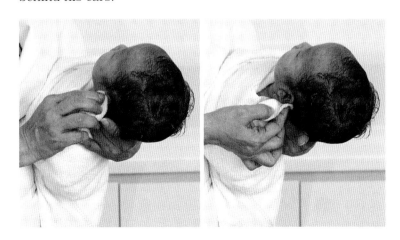

Cleaning Baby's Genital Area

Put your baby back on the protective sheet. Before removing the towel completely, use it to dab his head dry.

Remove the towel and his diaper. Use baby wipes to clean your baby's genital area, starting from the front to the back.

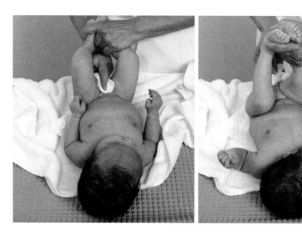

Putting Baby into the Bath

Support your baby's head, neck and shoulder with your left forearm and hold his upper left arm with your left hand.

Put your right arm under him and hold his left thigh with your right hand.

Gently lift your baby and lower him into the tub. Holding your baby securely under his armpit with your left hand, wash him with your right hand.

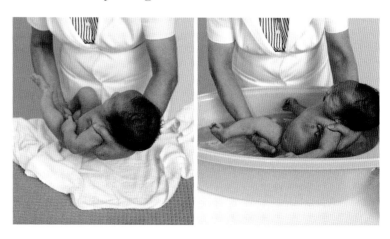

Washing Baby's Body

Wash the front of his body, arms, legs and the genital area. Then, lean him forward, supporting his chin on your right forearm and holding his left armpit securely with your right hand. Wash his back and buttocks with your left hand.

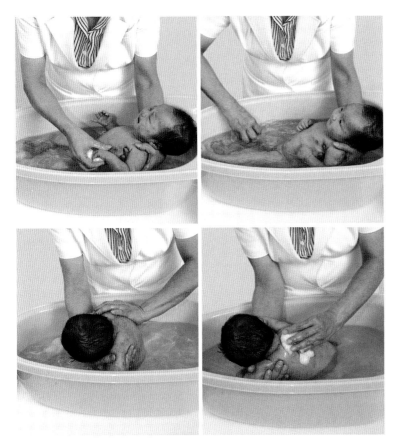

Drying Baby

When you are done, lift him out of the bath the same way you lifted him in and place him on a clean towel. Gently dab him dry. Be sure to dry behind his ears, between his fingers and toes, armpits, neck and groin area and any skin folds on his body.

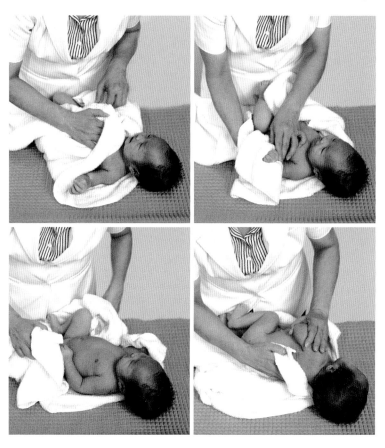

Dressing Baby

Put a fresh diaper on your baby and dress him. Mittens will help keep your baby warm and prevent him from scratching himself.

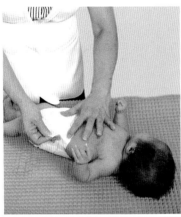

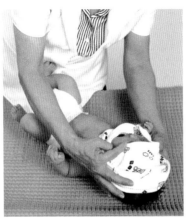

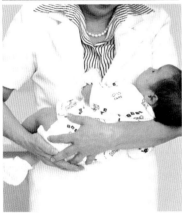

Using Diapers

Feeding and cleaning your baby will take up almost all of your time in the day and at night too. To keep your baby comfortable and happy, and to prevent rashes on his sensitive skin, keep him clean and dry. Should you use cloth or disposable diapers? The choice is yours. You can also choose to use both—cloth diapers at home and disposables for when you are on an outing or on holiday.

Cloth Diapers

Cloth diapers are not what they used to be. Some now come with Velcro-strips, making them easy to use without the need for big safety pins. Others are made of multi-ply fibre, which make them more absorbent.

The obvious advantage of cloth diapers is that they can be reused and are therefore cheaper in the long run.

Many parents also find that cloth diapers are less likely to cause diaper rash in their babies because they are made of natural cotton.

Disposable Diapers

Disposable diapers offer convenience. There is no need for laundering, making it a good option for outings or when you are travelling. Disposable diapers also leak less because they fit snugly. When using disposable diapers however, be sure to check the diaper often and replace it whenever it is wet or soiled.

Choosing the Right Disposable Diaper

With so many different diaper brands and variants, how do you choose what's best for your baby? The hospital where you will deliver your baby will provide a small pack of diapers for newborns and you can choose to continue with the same type of diapers if you find them suitable. As your baby grows, however, you will need to find new diapers for his changing needs. Here are some things to consider:

* Size. Diapers are categorised by weight of the baby so choose one that suits your baby's weight, not age.

* Material. Diapers made of soft, cloth-like material allow your baby's skin to breathe and will be more comfortable for your baby.

* Absorbency. Find out from friends which brand of diaper they find most absorbent and buy a small pack to try out first.

* Closure tabs. Some diapers come with resealable Velcro tabs, making it easy for you to check baby's diaper whenever you need to. The ones with adhesive tape might not work as well, especially if your hands are wet or greasy after moisturising your baby.

How Many Diapers?

It has been estimated that a baby will use up to 7,000 diapers from the time he is born till the time he becomes potty-trained.

Diaper Rash

Diaper rash is caused by continual exposure to dampness and the ammonia contained in urine. It is easily identified by the red patches and bumps on the genitals, buttocks and, in more severe cases, beyond the diaper area.

The best way to avoid diaper rash is to keep your baby's genital area clean and dry. Over-the-counter diaper rash creams containing zinc oxide can effectively prevent and cure mild to moderate cases of diaper rash. If possible, let your baby go without his diaper for a few hours during the day to clear up the rash.

Baby Massage

Massaging and touching your baby is a loving way to bond. Your gentle and comforting motions as you massage your baby will also help to soothe him and enable him to sleep better.

Massaging Your Baby

Just as an adult may enjoy and benefit from a full body massage, your baby will enjoy your loving touch as you take the time to gently massage him. Massage allows you to spend quiet moments with your baby and will help both of you to bond and relax.

Talk and sing to your baby as you massage him and tune in to the sounds and movements that he makes. If your baby smiles, coos, reaches out or looks at you, he is enjoying his massage. If he pulls away, frowns, starts being fussy or cries, stop the massage session and pick up your baby to comfort him. Massage can:

* Help relax your baby and ease any fussiness or irritability.

* Enable your baby to sleep more soundly and for longer as he is more relaxed.

* Enhance the bond between you and your baby.

* Make you more sensitive to your baby's cues and his body language.

Steps to a Simple Massage

A good time to massage your baby is after his bath or just before you put him to sleep. A 10-minute massage is sufficient for newborns. Increase this to 15 to 20 minutes for an older baby. Each stroke should be done about five or six times.

Start by massaging one leg, beginning from the pelvic joint
and moving down towards the ankle. Continue to massage
in the other direction, from the ankle towards the pelvic joint.

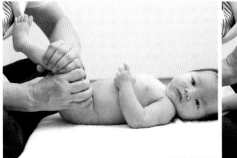 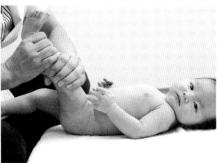

Gently squeeze each toe and massage the sole and the top
of the foot.

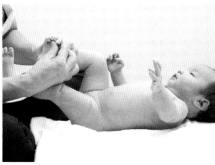 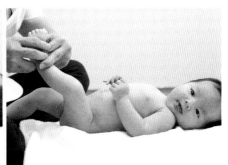

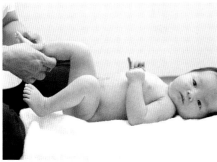

Repeat leg and foot massage on the other leg.

Stomach and Chest

Make a circle in a clockwise direction on your baby's stomach with the palm of one hand, simultaneously making a half-circle in a clockwise direction with your other hand.

Massage your baby's chest by gliding each palm diagonally across baby's chest, and then from the centre of baby's chest towards his sides and back to the centre in a heart-shaped motion.

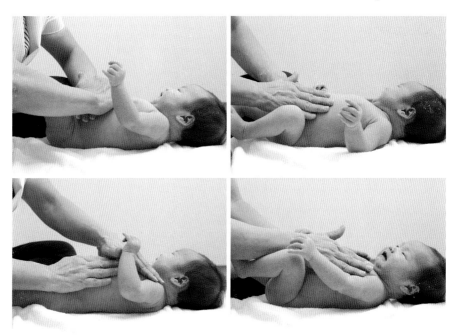

Arms and Wrists

Hold your baby's arm up and gently stroke it from the shoulder down towards the wrist. Continue to massage in the other direction, from the wrist towards the shoulder.

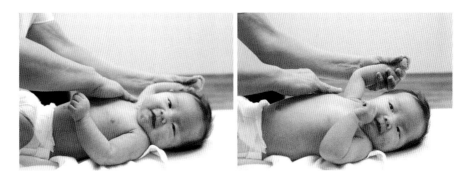

Gently massage your baby's wrist and hand. Repeat arm and wrist massage on the other hand.

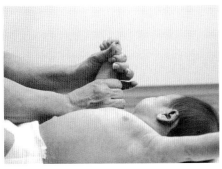 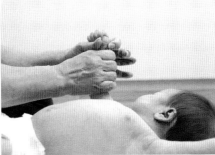

Face

Gently stroke baby's face with your thumbs, from his upper lips out towards his cheeks. Massage his jawline in circular motions, from his ears to the chin.

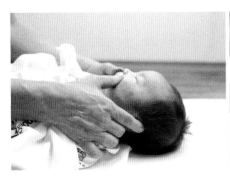 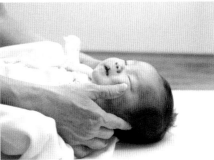

Back

Lie your baby on his stomach and stroke him from his neck down to his buttocks, using vertical and then horizontal strokes.

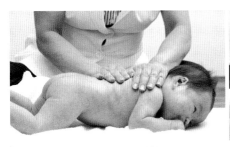 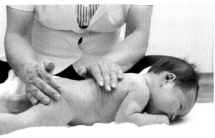

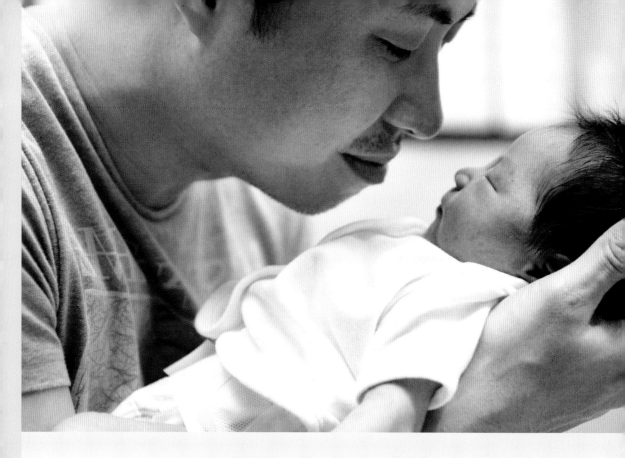

SPECIAL ROLE OF DADS

Gone are the days when it was thought that child rearing was a woman's job. Today, mums and dads share an equal role in raising their children. Many dads now enjoy a warm and close relationship with their children through playing, guiding, teaching and daily care-giving.

From the Start

Dads can start playing a supportive role while the baby is still in the womb, such as attending antenatal classes and going along for prenatal checkups with mum.

After the baby is born, dad can help with housework, cooking, changing diapers as well as looking after baby's older siblings if any to enable mum to have more time with the baby.

If dad is involved in the baby's care, the baby will soon recognise his face and be able to be comforted by him as well as by mum. In this way, mum can have some time to herself while dad and baby bond.

SPECIAL ROLE OF GRANDPARENTS

What children need most are what grandparents provide in abundance—unconditional love, kindness, patience, comfort and lessons in life. Your child's life will be much richer if he has a loving relationship with his grandparents.

However, grandparents are apt to spoil grandchildren and give advice. This can be a thorny issue, more so if you are living under the same roof. Here are some pointers for maintaining a good relationship with your parents and parents-in-law.

- ☐ Make them feel valuable. Giving you advice is a way of making themselves feel needed, so ask them for their advice sometimes. It will go a long way towards helping them feel that they are involved in their grandchild's life.

- ☐ Do not get defensive. It is natural to be defensive if you feel that they are judging you when they are simply sharing their experiences. Try to listen—you may learn something valuable.

- ☐ Pick your battles. If your mother or mother-in-law insists that both you and your baby stay home or avoid crowded air-conditioned places during his first few months of life, just bear with it and choose to go to places she would approve of. But stand your ground if it concerns the health or well-being of your child.

- ☐ Steer clear of sensitive topics. If your parents or parents-in-law insist that you give your baby formula to supplement breastfeeding because your baby looks too skinny, but you would prefer that your baby is fully breastfed, do not complain to them about how tiring breastfeeding is to avoid giving them the chance to bring up the topic. But should they bring up the topic, try to divert their attention and talk about something else.

- ☐ Quote your doctor. If your parents or parents-in-law insist that you start your baby on solids before you feel he is ready, speak to them nicely to help them understand that you are following your doctor's advice.

Asian Confinement Practices

Confinement practices vary from culture to culture. In Asia, these practices are based on the principles of yin and yang, and the belief that mothers lose a lot of heat after giving birth. As such, most Asian practices seek to help the mother conserve body heat and prevent chills.

The Confinement Month

This is an Asian custom whereby women who have just given birth are confined to the home for the first month. This period is a time for mums to rest and refrain from any heavy physical work. Apart from visits to the doctor, they are to avoid going outdoors especially at night, as it is believed that giving birth causes the mother's body to lose heat and she might catch a cold or become ill. Practices such as wearing socks and bedroom slippers, long clothing and not bathing are all attempts to prevent the body from losing heat. According to some old wives' tales, failure to keep to these confinement practices will mean suffering from health problems like rheumatism, headaches and other body pains later in life.

Different races have their own set of practices when it comes to confinement care but the objectives are largely similar—to help the mother recover from childbirth. Whether you decide to follow these practices or not, well-meaning family members and friends may offer you such advice. Take it in your stride.

What the Chinese Believe

* A confinement nanny will be able to take care of the mother by cooking special confinement food to help her rebuild her strength. The nanny will also be able to take care of the baby so the mother can rest and recover from the rigours of childbirth.

* Rheumatism and body aches experienced later in life are caused by washing hair, drinking cold water or bathing in cold water, having the fan or air conditioner on and consuming 'cooling' food during the confinement month.

* To avoid the negative effects of taking a shower, use only specially prepared warm water infused with herbs.

* Consuming special confinement food cooked with ginger and other traditional herbal tonics will keep the body warm, improve blood circulation and strengthen the joints weakened by childbirth.

* Consuming fish soup will boost milk supply.

What the Malays Believe

* A traditional Malay massage and wrap with herbal preparations and heat treatment with hot stones will help improve blood circulation, keep the body warm and return the body to its pre-pregnancy shape.

* Eating freshwater fish will promote healing internally.

* Eating mackerel, shellfish and prawns may cause allergies and itchiness.

* Drinking cold water and consuming 'cooling' food such as water spinach, cucumber and young coconuts are bad for blood circulation and will cause muscle aches and pains, rheumatism, arthritis and weak joints later in life.

What the Indians Believe

* Warm herbal baths will help improve blood circulation and reduce fatigue.

* Daily massages using special oil blends such as mustard seed or sesame seed oils will help the body recuperate after childbirth.

* Traditional Indian dishes like *harira* (a lentil soup) and *panjiri* (a sweet snack) will provide vital nutrients to help speed up recovery, cleanse the uterus and boost the production of breast milk.

* Increased consumption of ghee will help the body regain strength and aid muscle repair.

* 'Cooling' food such as cucumber, cabbage and pineapple can cause rheumatism and arthritis.

* If breastfeeding, eating 'windy' food such as onion and jackfruit may cause colic in the baby while eating seafood will cause the baby to develop a rash.

Preventing Back Pain

You will be surprised how much your back can hurt from taking care of your baby, even a newborn. Here are some tips for preventing back pain.

* Instead of stretching your arms out to pick up your baby, bring him close to your chest before lifting. Avoid twisting your body.

* To pick up your baby from the floor, bend at your knees and not at your waist.

* When getting your baby out of the crib, put the crib side down instead of bending over the crib and lifting your baby over the top.

* When breastfeeding, bring the baby to your breast rather than bending over your baby.

* Sit in an upright chair instead of a soft couch when nursing your baby.

* When strapping your baby into the car seat, kneel on the back seat as you place the baby into the car seat instead of doing it from outside the car.

Asian traditions take special care of the mother after delivery, which include adhering to a special confinement diet that features special ingredients such as chicken and ginger, which are considered 'warm', while forbidding items that are considered 'cold'. This is all in keeping with the belief that childbirth causes the mother to lose heat.

All this attention is not for nothing. Modern nutrition science has proven that a woman's nutrient needs are at the highest in her life just after delivery as she establishes breastfeeding. So, the best confinement diet aims to meet all the nutrient needs of the mother to support the volume and quality of milk production. Over-strict diets that limit many food types will compromise the health and nourishment of mother and child.

Tips when Breastfeeding

Stay Well Hydrated

Breast milk is over 87 percent water. Breast milk volume increases from a few millilitres in the first few days to as much as 700 ml or more weeks later to keep abreast of baby's demand. Many women experience increased thirst during breastfeeding and this is a natural driver to drink. While water hydrates, use this opportunity to also consume beverages such as maternal milk supplements, milk, yoghurt, milkshakes, fruit juices and soups that deliver many vital nutrients.

Eat More Food

You need to eat 500 kcal more each day if you are breastfeeding. This is quite a bit but not a lot! Use your extra energy allowance to get a variety of nutrients by including various food such as grains like rice, noodles and bread, especially wholegrain varieties; fruit; vegetables; lean protein such as chicken, fish and lean meat; beans, nuts and seeds; as well as non-fat milk and milk products.

Consume More Protein

Focus on getting 25 g more of protein each day to support the production of breast milk. Two glasses of milk and 45 g of meat or fish would virtually make up for the extra need.

Choose the Right Fats

Fifty percent of the calories of breast milk come from fat. Here is one time in life that you should aim to include the right fats in your diet each day. Select unsaturated fats, especially those that provide the essential fatty acids—docosahexaenoic acid (DHA) and arachadonic acid (AA)—as they play a critical role in the optimal development of baby's brain and eye. Two servings of fatty fish such as salmon, tuna and mackerel each week will provide the necessary DHA. AA is found in meat, poultry and eggs.

Ensure Adequate Intake of Minerals

The need for many minerals, especially iron, iodine and zinc, increases during this time. Calcium needs remain high. Poor maternal diets will drain your body's reserves.

Ensure Adequate Intake of Vitamins

Water soluble vitamins such as thiamin, riboflavin and vitamin C levels in breast milk improve when your diet includes these vital nutrients. Fresh fruit and vegetables, milk, cheese, lean meat, fish, nuts and seeds are all good sources of many vital vitamins.

Food to Avoid

As your nutrient needs are very high when breastfeeding, focus on eating clean and safe food to prevent an episode of diarrhoea and vomiting. Just as you did during pregnancy, avoid eating large fish in favour of smaller ones. Also, limit your caffeine intake to no more than 500 ml of coffee each day as this may help prevent restlessness in your baby.

Preparing Your Older Child

One of the events that often causes stress for a child is the arrival of a new baby. However, with some preparation you can help your older child accept and adjust to the new addition to the family.

Tips to Prepare Your Older Child

* Talk to your older child about the baby and let him feel the baby's movement in your womb.

* Involve him when you are preparing things for the new baby.

* Prepare him for when you have to be away for the birth of your baby. Reassure him about who will care for him then.

* Let him know what to expect of the new baby—that he will be little, will not able to play or wait for his feed and that he will cry and need to be carried.

* Talk to him about his own birth and when he was a baby. Read stories to him about having a new baby.

* Keep reassuring him that he will be equally loved and cared for as the new baby.

* Encourage him in his role as the older sibling.

Children's reactions to the arrival of a new baby vary and depend on their temperament, age and parents' behaviour. Young children do not quite grasp what is happening and have not reached a stage in their emotional development that allows them to control or express their feelings. So, it is common for the older child to show jealousy, to regress to baby behaviour or bedwetting and be clingy or deliberately naughty and aggressive when the new baby arrives, although not all do this.

For some, it takes a while to realise that their new brother or sister is a permanent fixture, and it is only later that their behaviour reflects the major change they have just experienced in their lives. Some children will ask pointedly when the baby is going back to the hospital.

More positive responses do occur as well. Children may be loving and show concern for their new baby, and by the time the new brother or sister is a year old, siblings have often developed a meaningful relationship, playing and spending time together.

Sibling Rivalry

The extent of jealousy that children feel over a brother or sister can take parents by surprise. This sibling rivalry cannot be prevented. It can be very trying and needs careful handling.

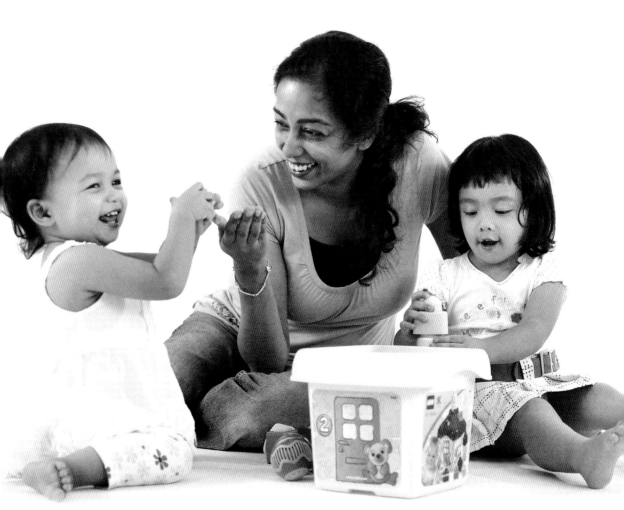

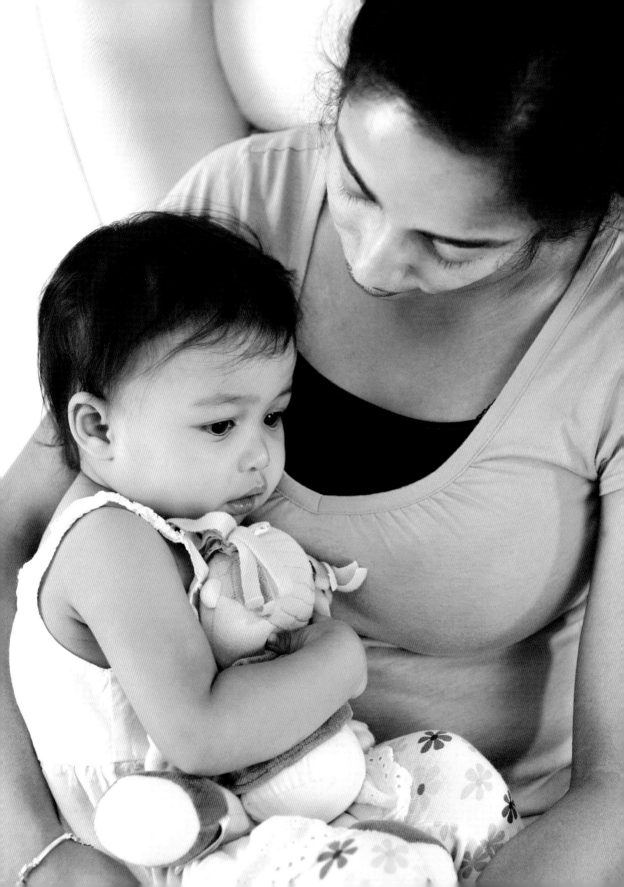

Your
Young Baby

Having made it through your baby's first month,
you are now more confident in handling him.
You would have found the best way to hold, comfort,
feed and dress him. Your baby will grow rapidly
in the first six months, doubling his birth weight
by the time he is 4 to 6 months old,
and trebling it by the time he is a year old.

Contributors:

Dr Chong Shang Chee
Ms Anna Jacob
Dr Jennifer Kiing
Dr Wendy Sinnathamby

| Pregnancy | 0 to 1 month | 2 to 11 months | 12 months to 3 years | 3 to 6 years |

Your Baby's Development

You will be amazed at how rapidly your baby will grow and develop in his first year. From a helpless newborn, he is likely to be toddling around by the time he turns one. Well before he is able to use language, he will be constantly making observations and connections about what is going on around him. By the time he is a year old, he will be able to say a few words although he is able to understand a whole lot more. Do not underestimate him!

Development Milestones

Your baby will be acquiring new skills rapidly throughout his first year, but the rate at which he develops will vary, so do not be overly concerned should he seem to be slower than other babies of the same age.

2 Months

Your baby will be able to recognise your face and smile in response when he sees you. He might also wave his arms in excitement and make gurgling noises.

Although his vision is still rather limited, he will be able to track nearby objects with his eyes, so tie activity quilts with colours and mirrors to the side of his cot and hang mobiles and chime toys above his cot to encourage him to reach out and explore.

Put your face close to his when you talk to him. This will also help you build a bond with your baby.

3 Months

Your baby will be able to raise his head and chest, and support his upper body with his arms when placed lying on his stomach.

He will become more aware of his hands and bring them to his mouth. To facilitate his hand-mouth coordination, place teething toys in his hands. Cloth toys and books will also encourage his grasping action. Place a rattle in his hand and show him how to shake it to produce sound.

4 Months

Your baby will have better control of his head and will be able to sit up with support. He will also be more curious about things around him and will turn his head in the direction of something that catches his attention. Prop him up with cushions so he can look around.

He will have better control of his hands and be able to bring them together and reach out for things more accurately. When placed lying on his back, he will bring his feet up and play with them. He will also begin rolling over, usually from his stomach to his back.

5 Months

Your baby will have full head control when pulled to a sitting position. He will be grabbing everything that is within reach so be careful not to place him near objects that could cause harm or injury.

His concentration is developing and he will spend more time examining toys and other objects.

You might also start to notice the emergence of first teeth on the front of the lower jaw.

6 Months

Your baby will be able to sit up without support for at least a few seconds. He will also raise his arms when he wants to be picked up. When he starts sitting up, give him toys that he can knock together, drop, put in and take out of containers and cause-effect toys involving push buttons and open-close mechanisms. Busy boxes, soft blocks, simple musical instruments, activity boards and pop-up toys are suitable. Fabric and cardboard picture books are also appropriate while large interlocking rings or keys promote manipulation.

He will open his mouth when you bring a spoon to his lips and may start showing interest in food that the family eats. These are signs that he is ready for complementary food.

He will start to babble and make sounds. Encourage the development of speech by singing to him and repeating rhymes.

7 Months

Your baby will be able to roll over both ways, from stomach to back and back to stomach, and will be starting to crawl. He is now able to support his weight on his legs and will enjoy being pulled to his feet.

He will make attempts to pick up small objects, perfecting his pincer grip and be able to press buttons.

He will begin to understand the meaning of words that you use often with him, such as "no", and will be able to locate objects that are partially hidden, demonstrating cognitive development. He will also begin to develop memory and look for toys he has dropped.

8 Months

Your baby will now be crawling steadily. He may be teething and start chewing on toys and other objects. Provide him with a chilled teething ring to soothe his gums.

He will recognise familiar songs, rhymes and games and turn his head when his name is called.

9 Months

Your baby is able to feed himself, picking up finger food with his thumb and index finger. Encourage him to master this skill by offering him cereal, baby biscuits and small pieces of fruit and vegetables.

He is able to say "mama" and "papa" and can associate words with their corresponding objects.

10 Months

Before he starts walking, your baby will 'cruise', pulling himself up on furniture and using it for support as he slides around it. Make sure you watch him or keep any unsteady furniture out of the way. Encourage him to walk by offering him your hands and pulling him up to a standing position.

He is able to transfer objects from hand to hand and drop toys with the intention of reaching for another.

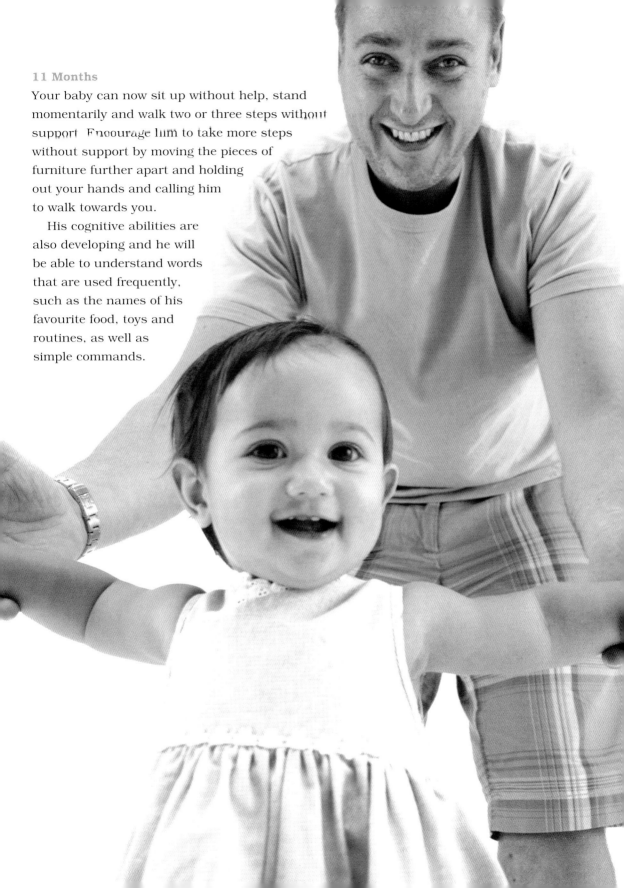

11 Months

Your baby can now sit up without help, stand momentarily and walk two or three steps without support. Encourage him to take more steps without support by moving the pieces of furniture further apart and holding out your hands and calling him to walk towards you.

His cognitive abilities are also developing and he will be able to understand words that are used frequently, such as the names of his favourite food, toys and routines, as well as simple commands.

Crying and Comforting

Crying is how babies express themselves. Check on your baby when he cries and see what he needs. He could be hungry, wet or just needing a cuddle. You are not spoiling him by picking him up when he cries. By responding to his cries promptly, he will learn to trust that someone will be there to meet his needs and feel loved. The longer he cries, the longer it will take to calm him down.

When Does the Crying Stop?

Be patient with your baby. Babies generally cry less as they get older, when they are about 4 to 5 months old.

Soothing Your Baby

Although babies usually cry because they are hungry, wet or uncomfortable, there will be times when your baby may cry for no apparent reason. Here are some tips to calm your baby down.

* Stay calm. If you are agitated, he will pick up on your vibes and cry even more.

* Hold your baby pressed against your chest and gently pat his back. With younger babies, swaddling may do the trick as it makes them feel snug and secure.

* Offer your baby a pacifier or teething ring if he is old enough to hold it in his hand. He may be experiencing teething pains.

* Sit in a rocking chair with your baby and rock back and forth. The rocking motion will help calm him down.

* Put him in the car or stroller or carry him and go for a walk. The movement may help calm your baby down.

* Talk or sing softly to your baby. Sometimes the soothing sound of your voice is all he needs to comfort him.

* Give your baby a massage to help loosen tense muscles.

* Put on some soft music. Sometimes even the whir of an electric fan or ticking of a clock can have a calming effect.

COLIC

When a healthy baby cries for prolonged periods, drawing up his legs and breaking wind, he is likely to be suffering from infantile colic. For first-time parents, this bout of recurrent, inconsolable crying can be worrying and nerve-wrecking.

Colic usually begins in the first few weeks after birth and lasts till the baby is about 3 months old. The main symptom is the sudden onset of regular and prolonged periods of crying which is believed to be caused by pain in the abdomen. This often occurs at the same time every day, usually in the evening.

While doctors still do not know the exact cause of colic in babies, they seem to think that it may be caused by the build-up of air in the stomach. To prevent your baby from swallowing more air, do not let him cry for too long before feeding him. If he is bottle-fed, tilt the bottle so that the milk covers the teat completely. Ensure that the hole in the teat is just right for your baby and not too big or too small. Whether breast- or bottle-fed, always burp your baby properly after his feed.

You can also try massaging your baby about an hour before the time when you expect him to start crying but not just after a feed. Move your hands clockwise in a gentle, circular motion over his stomach.

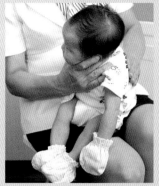

BURPING YOUR BABY

There are a few methods for burping your baby. Babies swallow air when they suck or cry and burping them helps to relieve wind and colic caused by swallowed air. If you are breastfeeding, burp him before breastfeeding and before giving the other breast. If bottle-feeding, burp him two or three times during the feed and at the end of the feed. Be patient. It sometimes takes a while for baby to burp.

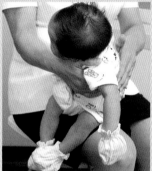

Method 1: Sit your baby upright on your lap. Support his chin or armpit and chest with one hand, or with your forearm, while gently patting his back with the other hand.

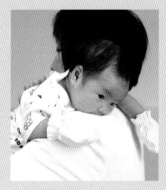

Method 2: Place your baby upright with his chin on your shoulder. Pat him gently on his back for 5 to 10 minutes.

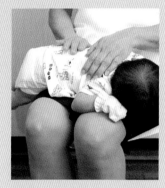

Method 3: Place your baby face down on your lap and pat his back for 5 to 10 minutes.

THE PACIFIER DILEMMA

Parents usually have a love-hate relationship with pacifiers. While they dislike seeing their baby with a pacifier, they love the fact that it soothes him when he is fretful.

Some Advantages of Using a Pacifier

- ☐ Pacifiers may help soothe a fussy baby. Most babies are contented when they are sucking on something. Pacifiers can help calm a baby when he is crying.

- ☐ Pacifiers may help your baby fall asleep. If he has trouble settling down, sucking on a pacifier might do the trick.

- ☐ Pacifiers can be taken away. Compared to sucking on his thumb or fingers, when it is time to wean your baby from the pacifier, you can take it away. It may be more difficult to break a thumb- or finger-sucking habit.

Some Disadvantages of Using a Pacifier

☐ Early pacifier use may interfere with breastfeeding. Some babies have trouble learning how to nurse properly if they are given a pacifier too soon.

☐ Your baby may become dependent on the pacifier. If your baby uses a pacifier to sleep, you may face frequent middle-of-the-night crying spells when the pacifier falls out of your baby's mouth.

☐ Prolonged pacifier use may cause a child's top front teeth to slant outward or not come in properly.

An appropriate time to wean your baby off the pacifier is before your baby's first birthday, when he starts babbling and/or teething.

Pacifier Dos and Don'ts

If you choose to offer your baby a pacifier, keep these tips in mind:

☐ Wait until breastfeeding is well established before you give your baby the pacifier.

☐ Do not pop a pacifier into your baby's mouth the minute he starts to fret or cry. See if he is hungry, tired or bored and try other ways of pacifying him before giving him the pacifier.

☐ If the pacifier falls out of your baby's mouth while he is sleeping, do not pop it back in.

☐ Sterilise the pacifier by putting it in boiling water for 5 minutes before first use. Make sure it is completely cooled down before giving it to your baby. Then, keep it clean by washing it in hot, soapy water and rinsing it well after each use.

☐ Replace pacifiers often and watch for signs of deterioration. A worn or cracked nipple can tear off and pose a choking hazard. Never use a string or strap long enough to get caught around your baby's neck.

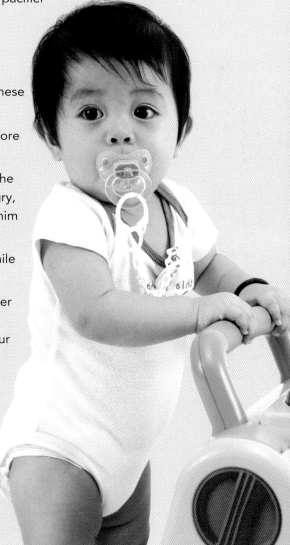

Introducing Solid Food

Some parents are eager to introduce their babies to the wonderful world of food that they themselves enjoy, but introducing solids too early poses a higher risk of baby developing food allergies later on. Do not let your baby start on solids until after 6 months. Before 4 months of age, his body is incapable of digesting and absorbing complex food. Instead, take your cue from your baby's changing feeding habits and developmental readiness. Here are some tips to make weaning a pleasant adventure for baby and you.

Probiotics and Prebiotics

Not all the bacteria in our digestive system are bad. While some can make us sick, there are those such as probiotics that are beneficial to us.

Probiotics are germs found in our large intestine and they have been shown to be advantageous in preventing infections such as gastroenteritis in children. They may also prevent the development of allergy during early childhood.

Prebiotics are non-digestible fibres that make their way through the digestive system and help the good bacteria to grow and flourish in the large intestine. Prebiotics are found naturally in breast milk.

Knowing when Baby Is Ready

You will know that your little one is ready when he shows interest in what other people around him are eating and when he opens his mouth when a spoon is brought near his lips. At this stage, your baby would have doubled his birth weight and can sit up with support.

Start with the Right Food

Soft rice porridge is one of the first items recommended as it is least likely to trigger an allergy. Ideally, an iron-fortified rice cereal is recommended as the first choice to prevent anaemia.

Once your baby has adapted to soft rice porridge, increase the variety to other grain food such as wheat and oats. Over the next few weeks, add vegetables and fruit followed by finely flaked boneless fish, finely minced cooked chicken and meat.

Hold back on fresh milk until baby is over a year old as it may trigger serious conditions such as faecal blood loss and low iron status. Fruit juices are best introduced diluted to prevent osmotic diarrhoea. Limit the consumption of juice to 125 ml each day when your baby is below a year old. You can then increase it to about 250 ml after this period.

Start with a Small Portion

The quantity to start with is about a teaspoonful. The aim of this small portion is to allow your baby to learn to eat. Once this basic function is established, the portion can be increased to meet your baby's nutritional needs.

From once a day, progress towards offering two or three small meals a day, in addition to his regular milk feeds. Meals of complementary food should be provided two or three times per day at 6 to 8 months of age and three or four times per day at 9 to 11 months and 12 to 24 months of age, with additional nutritious snacks offered once or twice per day, as desired.

Introduce One Food at a Time

This practical tip is to help you identify any food that your baby may not tolerate well or is allergic to. Once a food is introduced to baby's menu, offer it for three days in a row. Be observant. If there seems to be no rashes or digestive disturbances, continue to offer another new food. Over time, your baby will have a variety of well-tolerated items to enjoy. If you or your family members have food allergies, it is best to introduce those potential allergens only after your baby is a year old.

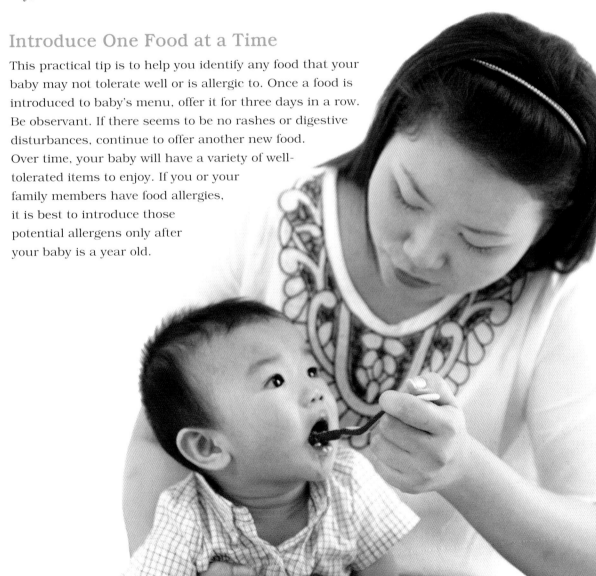

Ensure the Right Texture

A baby's ability to swallow and chew is limited so start with food that is smooth and runny. As your baby becomes more adept at handling food, change the texture from runny to finely minced and even soft food before introducing more lumpy food. One school of thought suggests that lumpy food should be introduced by 9 months of age or the baby will be likely to refuse texture variations.

Deliver Food Safely

Ensure that your baby is supervised at every feeding time. All food and drink must be prepared hygienically. Serve food warm but not hot and avoid food items that are hard to chew, swallow or include slippery peels and seeds or bones.

Encourage Self-feeding

As your baby grows, he will show interest in feeding himself by indicating that he wants to hold the spoon or touch the food. Encourage this as it will help him to learn to eat independently. While he may at times want to play with the food, do not keep the spoon away from him, but be firm with him and show him how he should be feeding himself. If he seems more interested in playing with the food, you can feed him in between his attempts.

While the mess that your baby creates may be a deterrent to allowing him to self-feed, do not be tempted to take over the feeding. Find a way around it. Try placing his high chair over some old newspapers or a mat and let him wear a bib. This will help you clean up in a jiffy while your baby gets the opportunity to learn to self-feed.

Introduce Family Food

After your baby's first birthday, you can start introducing him to age-appropriate food from the family table. This will help him to adapt to the family menu early.

FREQUENTLY ASKED QUESTIONS

Why does my baby spit out the food?
Relax, your baby is not protesting against your cooking skills! In the first 4 months, the tongue thrust reflex protects the infant against choking. When any unusual substance is placed on the tongue, it automatically protrudes outwards rather than back. By the time he is 6 months old, an infant can voluntarily control suckling and swallowing, and biting movements will begin. The tendency to push solids out of the mouth also decreases. So if your baby seems to be spitting out food, wait a week or so and try again.

What should I do when my baby rejects a particular food?
Most food preferences are learnt and acquired early in life. Liking an unfamiliar food can be encouraged by increasing his exposure to the food. So do not give up. Try and try again.

What if my baby does not want to eat the food prepared?
Your initial goal in feeding is to introduce your baby to the new tastes and textures of solid food, not to give him a whole meal. Never force-feed your baby. If he is not keen to eat, offer him food later in the day.

There are many reasons why your baby may not be ready to eat. Here's how you can figure that out:

- Your baby purses his lips and turns his head away from the approaching spoon.

- Your baby seems uninterested or wants to avoid the food.

Is commercial baby food nutritious?
While most mothers like to prepare fresh food from scratch for their babies, commercial baby food is a convenient choice. In general, most commercial baby food delivers valuable nutrients in fair amounts and do not include sugar, salt and other food additives. So while you can prepare baby food at home with ease, do not feel guilty if you do open a jar of commercial baby food when needed. Pick a product that offers a variety of textures that suit your baby's eating ability.

Weaning

You can continue breastfeeding for as long as both you and your baby desire. There is no need to wean your baby from your breast but some babies gradually lose their desire to suckle when they start on solid food.

Reasons for Weaning

There are many reasons why mothers wean their babies off the breast, and these include returning to work, wanting more time for themselves and pressure from family.

If your reason for weaning is because you are returning to work, a good solution is to express your breast milk (page 96) at work so your baby can be fed using the bottle in the day and resume suckling when you return home.

If you are pressured to wean by family members, try explaining the benefits of breastfeeding (page 91) to them. This is a decision you should make for yourself and your baby, so persevere if your desire is to continue breastfeeding.

If you feel that the time has come for you to wean your baby, here are some tips to help you along.

Make the Switch Gradually

Eliminate one feed every few days to allow your milk supply to decrease gradually. After a couple of weeks, you should be nursing just a couple of times a day. Usually the last feeds to go are the first one in the morning and the last one at night.

Let Someone Else Give the Bottle

If you have been nursing your baby since birth, he will associate you with breastfeeding and may be confused or upset if that changes. Try letting a family member give him the first few bottles of expressed breast milk or formula milk while you stay out of sight. After he gets used to the bottle, you can take over.

Head Straight to the Cup

If your child is older than a year, skip the bottle and introduce a sippy cup as you wean him off the breast.

Expect Some Engorgement

Once you stop breastfeeding completely, your milk production will stop fairly quickly. In the meantime, you may need to express some milk for the first few days to avoid engorgement. But do not express so much that you stimulate milk production. To ease the discomfort, apply cold compresses and take a mild pain reliever if needed.

Make It Stress-free

To make weaning as stress-free as possible for yourself and your baby, take it easy and do it gradually. Do not get upset if you backslide. Just get back on track again.

Formula Milk or Cow's Milk

Until your baby is about a year old, his digestive tract is not developed enough to process the complex proteins present in cow's milk. So if you wean your baby before then, give him formula milk as this contains the vital nutrients that he requires for optimal growth.

Research has shown that children have an increased risk of developing allergic conditions such as asthma and eczema, and diabetes (especially if there is a family history of it), if started on cow's milk before they are a year old.

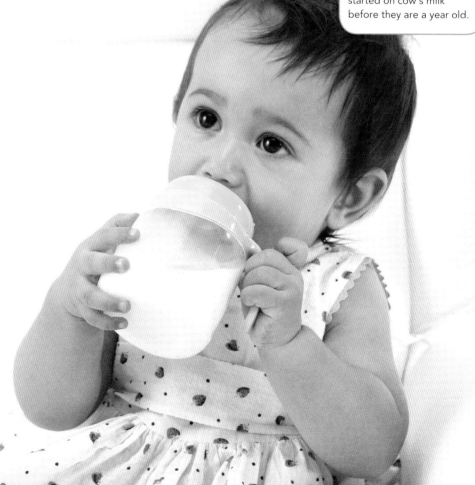

Oral Health

Having strong and healthy teeth is important for your child's overall health and well-being. Oral care can begin in the first few days of life, with you wiping your baby's gums with a clean piece of gauze or small towel to remove plaque. Once his teeth come through, you can begin brushing them with a soft toothbrush and water. The important thing is to get your child used to brushing his teeth as part of his daily routine.

Teething

Some children start teething at around 5 to 8 months of age, while others may not develop teeth until they are more than a year old. Your child will have his full set of milk teeth or baby teeth by the time he is about 2½ years old.

Soothing the Gums

If your baby's gums look sore and red, and your child gnaws at his toys, it might be due to teething. Here's what you can do to provide your child with some relief.

* Gently rub his gums with a clean finger, a small, cool spoon or a wet gauze pad.

* Give him a clean teething ring to chew on. Chilling it in the refrigerator beforehand may help.

Preventing Tooth Decay

As soon as teeth appear in your baby's mouth, tooth decay can occur so it is important that you help your child to care for his teeth.

* When bottle-feeding, give only plain milk or water and not juices or sweetened drinks.

* Do not let your baby fall asleep with the bottle.

* If you use a pacifier, make sure that it is clean.

* Never dip the pacifier in sugar or honey before giving it to your child.

* Make brushing teeth a fun activity. Let your child watch you brush your teeth, then give him a small toothbrush to imitate you. While he may want to brush his teeth himself, he will not have the dexterity to clean them properly before he is 5 or 6 years old. Follow up by brushing them for him.

* When your child is around 2 years old, start brushing his teeth with a pea-sized amount of toothpaste. There are toothpastes especially for children in different flavours. Show him how to rinse his mouth with water and then spit it out.

First Visit to the Dentist

You should take your child for his first dental checkup when he is a year old and not later than 2½ years old when he has all his milk teeth. Fear of the dentist is not inborn. It is something he learns from a bad experience or hearing about unpleasant experiences from others.

Preparing Your Child

* Help your child prepare for his first visit by playing "at dentist" at home with him. Talk about what to expect on his visit.

* Take him with you when you go for your dental checkup.

* Make the appointment at a time of day when your child is not tired. On the day of the appointment, give yourself plenty of time to get ready. Be relaxed yourself so that you do not communicate your anxiety to your child and make him tense.

* Do not make the dentist the villain— someone you will take him to if he does not brush his teeth or when he misbehaves!

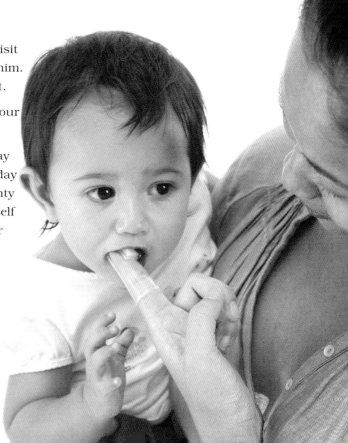

Going Out

Take your baby out to enjoy interesting sights and sounds whenever you can and help him to develop and learn. Babies already have a sense of touch, smell and taste at this age, and are developing sight and hearing. Start with a family day out or even just a quick visit to the store.

Sun Protection

Take care to protect your baby's skin from sun damage. UV rays from the sun can cause burns and contribute to the development of skin cancer later in life.

If your baby is 6 months and younger, it is best to keep him out of the sun. If you have to take him out, minimise his exposure to the sun with protective clothing and a hat, and use an umbrella or mesh cover over his stroller. When your baby is older, keep him well-protected from the sun with:

* Hats. Choose sun hats with wide brims that shield the face as well as the neck.

* Sunglasses. Check that the lenses provide full protection against UVA and UVB rays. Some sunglasses for children come with a sports band to hold the glasses in place.

* Sunscreen. Apply one that offers protection against both UVA and UVB rays and a sun protection factor (SPF) of at least 30. Apply it liberally every two hours that your baby is in the sun.

Baby Strollers and Carriers

Baby strollers and carriers offer convenience so you do not have to be cradling your baby in your arms all the time. Baby carriers are great for short trips while baby strollers will allow your baby to sit or lie down on longer outings.

Baby Strollers

The wide variety of baby strollers available can overwhelm new parents. Just what should you look for in a baby stroller?

* Buckles that lock securely and yet are easy to latch and unlatch. The harness should fit snugly and comfortably around your baby's waist and there should be crotch straps to prevent baby from sliding down.

* Adjustable seat. A fully reclining seat is recommended for newborns. This feature is also suitable for your young baby who may need to nap while you are out.

* A stroller with a sun shield will protect your child from the sun and rain.

* A removable seat made of washable fabric so you can keep the stroller clean and hygienic.

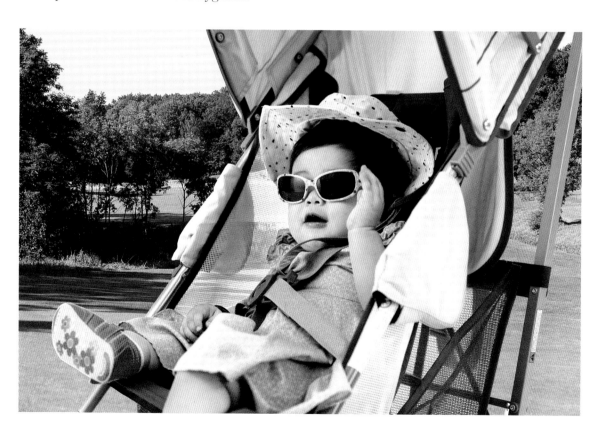

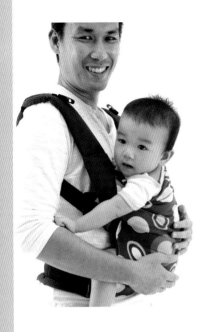

* Wheels that lock in place, a wheel base that is wide for stability and wheels that swivel for easy manoeuvrability.

* Ease of use. The stroller should ideally allow you to operate it with one hand, leaving the other hand free to hold your baby.

* Portability. The stroller should fit your lifestyle—light enough for carrying around if you use public transport and small enough to fit into the boot of a taxi or your car.

Baby Carriers

A baby carrier is ideal for keeping a tiny baby where he is happiest—close to your body so he is reassured by your heartbeat and can enjoy the rhythm of your movements. It also frees your hands for other tasks. Here are some points to consider when getting a baby carrier.

* Weight allowance. Some carriers are made for babies weighing up to 14 kg (about 2 years old), while some are only suitable for newborns.

* Comfort for you. Carriers with wide shoulder straps will allow for more even weight distribution over your back and shoulders.

* Comfort for baby. The carrier should provide good support for your baby's head and back.

* Flexibility of carrying positions. Choose a carrier that allows baby to face inwards or outwards so you can adjust the position to suit your baby's moods and preferences.

* Ease of use. The carrier should be easy to put on and take off without assistance. It should also pack away neatly into your baby bag.

* Material. A carrier made of lightweight, breathable fabric is suitable for warm climates, especially if you will be using it for long periods of time. Check that it is washable and can dry quickly after washing.

It is a good idea to try out a few carriers with your baby before you finally decide which one is most comfortable for you and your baby.

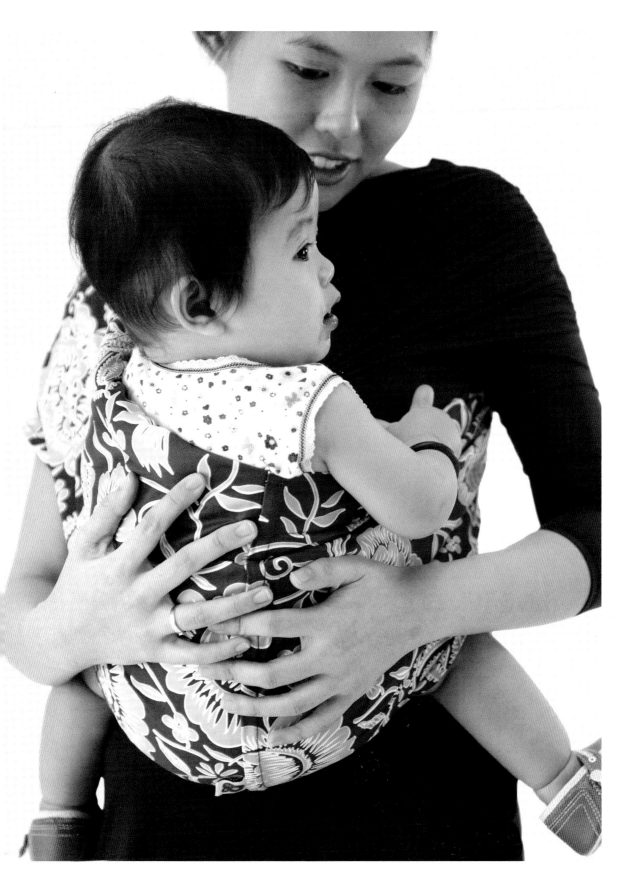

Travelling

Whether it is a road trip to a nearby destination or a long haul flight halfway across the world, travelling with children presents unique challenges. With some planning and preparation however, you can make it an enjoyable experience for the whole family.

Getting Ready to Go

Get Vaccinated

For a trip abroad, schedule a visit to your doctor six to eight weeks before leaving. Inform your doctor of your travel plans and he will be able to advise you on immunisation requirements. Some vaccines may require a period of time before the immunity is achieved.

Pack a First Aid Kit

Ask your doctor or pharmacist for medication for colds, fever and diarrhoea that is suitable for your child. Put these into a first aid kit with plasters, a thermometer and nail clipper. Depending on your destination, you may also want to include insect repellent, bug-bite lotion and sunscreen.

Include Essentials

Two weeks before you leave, make a list of the things you need for your child such as milk formula, diapers and feeding equipment, and remember to pack them. Do not forget to include some favourite snacks and toys or games to keep him occupied.

Time Your Trip

Plan your travel to coincide with your child's normal sleeping time. This will be less unsettling for him as he will be rested on arrival at your destination.

On the Flight

Dealing with Air Pressure

If travelling by air, your child may experience ear pain during take-off and landing due to the change in air pressure. To prevent this, breastfeed or offer a milk bottle or pacifier to your young baby. For an older child, give him a sweet to suck on.

Keeping Hydrated

It can be dehydrating on a plane so offer your children lots of fluid throughout the length of the journey.

Warming up Baby's Food

If you get the flight attendants to warm up food for you, they may use a microwave oven. As microwave ovens tend to heat up food unevenly, stir the heated food well and check the temperature before giving it to your child.

At Your Destination

Keeping Healthy

Dehydration from traveller's diarrhoea can be dangerous in children under 2 years old. Avoid offering your child salads and raw seafood and give him only well-cooked food.

Assume that all local water supplies and ice are unsafe even for brushing your teeth. Buy bottled water or boil water before using or drinking. Make sure all milk products have been boiled or pasteurised.

Dealing with Jet Lag

Give yourself some time to get over any jet lag. As far as possible, try to keep to the day and night at your destination by keeping your child active and not letting him take long naps during the day. This will enable him to sleep well at bedtime.

Returning to Work

For some women, returning to work is a heart-wrenching affair. How do you deal with the emotional upheaval of leaving your baby and going back to the working world again? It's not going to be easy but preparing yourself early will make the transition less stressful on you and your baby.

Let Go of the Guilt

You should not feel guilty about going back to work. For some women, the interaction and challenges at work make them better mothers than if they were to stay home feeling tied down and dissatisfied.

Making Arrangements

Dependable Child Care

If you are getting a live-in domestic helper, have the helper come in at least a month before you go back to work. This will give you sufficient time to train her as well as see if she is able to take good care of your baby. Ideally, have a family member check in on the helper to see how she is coping in the first week after you have gone back to work.

If you are leaving your baby with his grandparents or in a child care facility, start one to two weeks earlier to get him familiar with the child minders and the place.

Speak to Your Boss

Increasingly, companies are looking into flexible work arrangements for mothers of young children. You may want to check if you can work part-time, flexi-time or from home. If your job requires frequent travelling, you may want to speak with your boss about holding off such trips while your baby is still young.

Change Your Nursing Schedule

About two weeks before returning to work, change the timing of your nursing schedule to fit in with your working hours. Check with your office about where you can express your milk during your working hours.

Return to Work in the Middle of the Week

It is a good idea to make arrangements such that your first day back at work is in the middle of the week. This way, you will have a few days to adapt before having to make it through a full week the following Monday.

Organise Your Time

Juggling work and a baby will be tough, as both demand all your time and attention. Try making daily to do lists— one for things to do at home and the other for things to do at work so you can organise your time. Do not feel bad if you need to ask for help from your spouse, family members or colleagues.

Stay Connected

Put a favourite photograph of your baby on your desk. Make phone calls to home or the child care facility to find out how your baby is doing. Get them to put the phone to your baby's ear so he can hear your voice. Spend some quality time with your baby when you get home.

Have a Back-up Plan

Plan ahead for occasions when you might have to look for alternative solutions to child care, such as when your child minder falls ill or has an emergency at home. Are you able to take time off or have someone step in to take care of your baby?

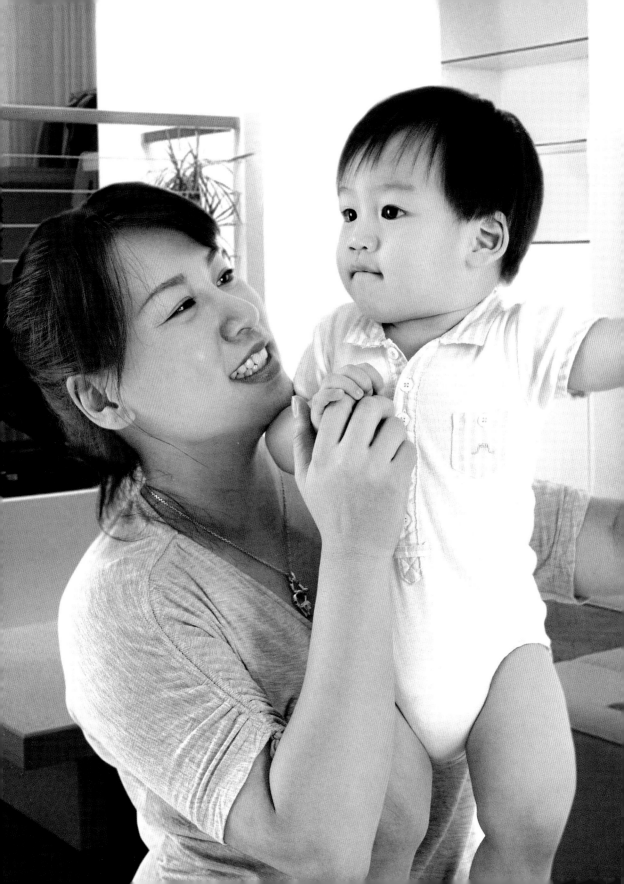

Your
Toddler

As your toddler begins to enjoy his mobility,
you will be kept on your toes running after him,
making sure he does not get himself into any dangerous
situations. He is also beginning to express himself and
may get into a temper tantrum when he thinks he is not
understood. This is one of the most challenging
periods and may leave you not knowing what to do. This
chapter will help you better understand your
toddler and take each situation in your stride.

Contributors:

Dr Chong Shang Chee
Ms Anna Jacob
Dr Jennifer Kiing

| Pregnancy | 0 to 1 month | 2 to 11 months | 12 months to 3 years | 3 to 6 years |

Your Toddler's Development

You and your toddler can have lots of fun developing his fine and gross motor skills through play. Give him old magazines to shred up and plastic containers of different sizes for water and sand play. To help him develop his speech and vocabulary, talk to him as much as possible. You will be amazed at how quickly he picks up language and be amused by some of the things he says. For many parents, seeing the world through the eyes of their children at this stage is an enlightening experience—one of the best things about being a parent!

Clumsy Children

Many children are clumsy during early childhood and most will grow out of it. But for some children, this clumsiness may persist and they will have difficulty throwing and catching a ball, managing the buttons on their clothes and find it hard organising things in sequence, such as which item of clothing to put on first. This may be due to their lack of perceptual motor skills which involve the coordination of sight and movement.

If you suspect your child has these difficulties (and they are more common in boys), take your child for an eye test first, then talk to your doctor. If necessary, get a referral to an occupational therapist or physiotherapist. Children who are clumsy can be shunned by other children and become lonely and disturbed if not given help.

Development Milestones

All children go through the same stages of development, with some developing a little earlier or later than others. As your child grows, he will become more proficient in his skills. Take note however that proficiency depends not only on maturation but also on the opportunities to use these skills and the encouragement given to develop them.

12 to 14 Months

Your young toddler will enjoy exploring objects by shaking, banging, throwing and dropping them. If you hide an object from him, he will be able to find it easily.

He will also enjoy imitating your gestures and can hold and drink from a cup, press the buttons on a telephone and put the receiver to his ear. If you have been reading and talking with him, he should be able to look at the correct picture in a book when the image is named and understand simple commands.

15 to 18 Months

Your toddler will be able to build a tower of two or three blocks, put two correct shapes into shape sorters, hold a crayon in his fist and open and close doors. He will also be able to point to parts of the body when asked.

19 to 24 Months

Your toddler will be able to walk steadily without help. With his new mobility, he will enjoy pulling toys behind him while walking, and carrying a large toy or several toys while walking. He will be starting to run and can stand on tiptoe. He will enjoy kicking balls and climbing up and down furniture. He can walk up and down stairs holding on to the banister and will put both feet on each step before moving on to the next step.

Your toddler will enjoy making circular scribbles and drawing vertical lines using crayons or colour pencils. He will also be able to build a tower of four to six blocks and turn the pages of books by himself.

He will be able to sort objects by shape and colour, and will begin make-believe play.

2 to 3 Years

Your toddler will be able to walk up and down stairs using alternate feet, run, hop, climb, pedal a tricycle and bend over without falling. He will be able to kick and throw a ball but will still have trouble catching a ball.

He will be able to remove a lid from a screw bottle, button and unbutton his clothes and thread string through beads. He will be able to hold a pencil steadily, although his grip will not be mature, and draw circles. He will be able to use scissors to cut paper.

He will know how to make mechanical toys work, sort objects by shape and colour and complete puzzles with three or four pieces. He will be able to match an object in his hand or in the room to a picture in a book and will enjoy playing make-believe with his toys, household pets and family members.

He will be able to understand and follow simple directions, as well as simple "When", "What", "Where", "Who" and "Why" questions. He will gradually stop referring to himself by name and start using pronouns such as "I", "me" and "you". He will be able to construct simple sentences that contain the important words to convey meaning while leaving the little words out.

Fitting the Pieces Together

Childhood, from birth to the age of 3, is a fascinating period. The way in which you respond to your child at this stage in his life will have a crucial impact on his ability to absorb new knowledge, think and reason about the world.

Around the age of 2, your child will begin to piece together all the fragments of information he has gathered about the world as a result of all his experiences. He will gradually accommodate or adjust his thinking to take on board these new ideas which he will store in his memory to retrieve when necessary.

Temper Tantrums

All children go through a phase when they throw temper tantrums, some more often than others. It may seem that your toddler is testing your patience, but the fact is that he does not enjoy throwing a tantrum anymore than you enjoy dealing with it.

Understanding Temper Tantrums

Tantrums are common when children are around 2 years old, a time when they are learning to talk. Because of their limited vocabulary, they have difficulty expressing themselves in words. As a result, they get frustrated when they are not understood and this may cause them to throw a tantrum. This is why this stage is often referred to as the "Terrible Twos". As children learn to express themselves better, the tantrums will decrease.

Reasons for Temper Tantrums

Tantrums run the gamut, from mild crying to bawling and rolling on the floor, kicking, screaming, vomiting and sometimes physically hitting out at the people around them. In order to help your toddler manage his emotional outbursts, understand what caused them in the first place. Below is list of possible reasons for a toddler throwing a temper tantrum.

* He may be tired from lack of rest or sleep.

* He may be thirsty or hungry.

* The environment at home may be unsettling. Is there a new member in the family, such as a new baby or a new helper? Are you and your spouse always quarrelling?

* He is unable to express verbally that he is angry or disappointed.

* He may be trying to get your attention.

* He wants to be independent and make his own decisions even at this young age.

* He may be frustrated because he is unable to accomplish a task that is too difficult.

* He may be feeling hot and bothered because of the weather or the clothes that he is wearing.

* You are not giving in to his demands.

Keeping Your Cool

Much as you may be driven to the edge, you should keep yourself in check and deal with your child's tantrums calmly. Even in the midst of his tantrum, he is unconsciously learning from you how to manage his emotions.

* You may reprimand him and make it known to him that this is unacceptable behaviour. But do not punish him because he might hold his anger and frustration inside, which can be unhealthy. Soothe him as best as you can and let him know that you understand his feelings.

* Ignore his tantrum if he is doing it because you did not give in to him.

* Do not fight his temper with your temper. You should not resort to physical punishment or yelling. Show him by example how to be calm and reasonable.

* Never offer him a bribe to stop his tantrum. This will only encourage him to throw tantrums when he wants his way.

* Distract him by doing something fun to defuse the situation, such as taking him outside to play or reading him his favourite story.

Tantrum Prevention

While you may not be able to stop his temper tantrums altogether, there are some things you can do to prevent them from happening too often.

Time Out

Time out is a discipline technique that will work with children from 2 years old, as they are old enough to understand the concepts of "waiting" and "being quiet". To learn more about using this technique to deal with your toddler's temper tantrum, turn to page 253.

* Avoid putting your toddler in stressful situations.

* Remove the potential triggers.

* Distract your toddler when you see that he is about to throw a tantrum.

* See that your toddler gets enough rest and sleep.

* Make sure that you have nutritious snacks readily available for when your toddler is feeling hungry between meals.

* Avoid major disruptions to your toddler's daily routine.

* Allow your toddler to make simple decisions for himself, such as whether he wants you to read a story to him or go out and play.

The good news is that tantrums should go away by the time your child is 4 or 5 years old. If they persist, you should consult your doctor to see if there is a serious behavioural or emotional problem and take steps to deal with it while he is still young.

Discipline with Love

The best way to teach your child discipline is with love. Harsh methods are not only ineffective in the long run, but your child may become resentful and rebellious.

* Keep your cool. Do not overreact by losing your temper or worse, spanking him when he makes a mistake or misbehaves. Talk to him calmly and explain why he should not do what he did. If you find yourself losing your cool, walk away and then deal with it when you have regained your composure.

* Do not over-praise. Going overboard with your praises makes them less meaningful and your child will start to wonder if you are sincere.

* Focus on your child's good points. He is more likely to heed what you say if you focus on what he is doing right rather than what he is doing wrong.

* Avoid physical punishment. Do not spank or cane your child. Try to discipline your child with love rather than fear.

* Reward good behaviour. Rewards need not and should not be only material things. It can be an extra story at bedtime to motivate your child to be on his best behaviour.

* Be a good role model. If you want your child to be kind and to respect others, you have to do the same yourself.

* Give unconditional love. Do not say things like "I don't love you because you're naughty." Make sure your child understands that it is the misbehaviour that you are unhappy with, not him, and that you will always love him.

Raising a Happy and Confident Child

Ideally, a child's main caregivers should be his parents. But when both parents are working, children are often left in the care of a domestic helper and/or grandparents. In this situation, as long as the adult taking care of your child is sensitive, perceptive and effective in meeting your child's needs, and your child is attached to the caregiver, your child will feel emotionally secure. Children who are emotionally secure are more likely to grow up happy and confident.

You need not lose out on the bonding and attachment with your child even if you are working. Give your child hugs and kisses before you leave for work. When you get home in the evening, spend time playing and reading with him and show interest in the things that he is doing.

As far as possible, try not to change domestic helpers too frequently. It is not uncommon to see children having behavioural problems when the helper whom they are attached to and who has been with them for a significant length of time leaves and is replaced by someone new. Children need consistency to feel secure.

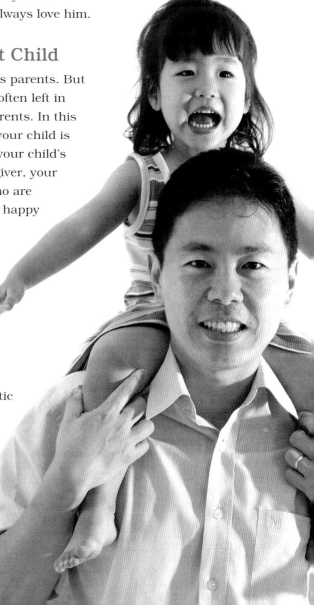

Food and Nutrition

The toddler stage from 1 to 3 years continues to be a period of rapid growth, with the first year being the most rapid. Your toddler's energy needs are high as he is more active, but his stomach is still small relative to his nutrient needs so provide him with food that is nutrient dense.

Variety Is the Key

Serve up a varied diet each day, made up of choices from each of the food groups represented in the Healthy Diet Pyramid—grains, fruit, vegetables, milk and milk products as well as meat and alternatives. Offer wholesome choices for meals and snacks. Do not force-feed your toddler but encourage him to have a healthy attitude towards food and eating.

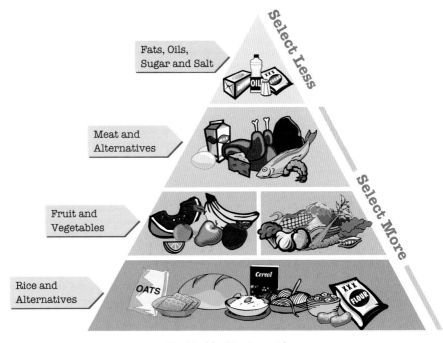

The Healthy Diet Pyramid

Milk Is a Must

Your toddler should consume milk or other dairy products two or three times daily. Fortified cow's milk is an important dietary component of a toddler's diet because of its high-quality protein, calcium, and vitamins A and D.

Limit Juices and Sweetened Beverages

If your toddler is thirsty, offer plain water. Limit your toddler's consumption of juice and sweetened beverages to no more than 180 ml daily.

Snacking Is Fine

As toddlers have small tummies, they are unable to eat enough at mealtimes to meet many nutrient goals. Help your toddler achieve his daily nutrient requirement by offering him nutritious snacks in between meals. Food from two of the four food groups should be offered for snacks, such as sandwiches and fruit, and meals should be made up of three of the four groups, such as rice, meat and vegetables.

Moderate Fat and Cholesterol

Do not restrict fat and cholesterol intake in your toddler's diet until he is at least 2 years old. After this age, fat should account for 25 to 30 percent of your toddler's total daily calories, with an emphasis on polyunsaturated fats.

Model Good Eating Behaviour

Children learn best when they see parents demonstrating the ideal behaviour. So model healthy eating and your toddler will soon eat right. Good nutritional habits should be fostered by sitting at the dining table, turning off the television and interacting as a family. Get your toddler involved, where possible, in the preparation of the food, such as going grocery shopping, washing vegetables or setting the table, and allowing him to watch you cook, then enjoying your meals together, as often as you can. This will go far towards helping your toddler improve the food choices that he will make later in life.

Picky Eating

Some children take to food and eating without much fuss. Others are simply difficult to feed. If your child is picky, you are not alone. In Singapore, 40 to 60 percent of parents think that their child is a picky eater.

Impact of Picky Eating

Some believe that picky eating is just a fad that lasts for a few days. But, with some children, feeding is a struggle that goes on and on for years.

Prolonged picky eating will affect the nutritional intake of the child and this will have a negative impact on his physical growth as well as mental performance over time.

Constant mealtime struggles will also impair the parent-child relationship. So if you are worried about your child's eating habits, talk with your doctor and he will be able to diagnose and treat the feeding difficulty.

Food Rules for Picky Eaters

You can also help your child overcome this by setting a few rules about food and eating.

* Avoid distractions. Do not allow toys, books, television or other distractions during meals or snacks.

* Maintain a neutral attitude. Praise your child for his self-feeding skills but keep a neutral attitude about his food intake.

* Do not use food as a present or reward, for comfort or as an expression of your affection.

* Feed to encourage appetite. Feed your child at regular times and space meals and snacks three to four hours apart. Offer water between meals and snacks.

* Limit the duration of mealtimes. End meals after 20 to 30 minutes, even if your child has eaten very little or nothing.

* Serve age-appropriate food and portions. Keep portions small and allow your child to ask for additional helpings.

* Encourage independent feeding and tolerate age-appropriate mess.

* Instil table discipline. Discourage your child from playing with his food and talking too much instead of eating. Teach him to sit at the table until everyone else has finished eating. Give one warning for misbehaviour, such as getting out of the chair or throwing food or utensils, followed by time out if the misbehaviour continues.

* Introduce new food systematically. Provide an appropriate complete and balanced nutritional supplement through this phase to ensure that your child is getting all the nutrients needed as he learns to overcome his feeding difficulty.

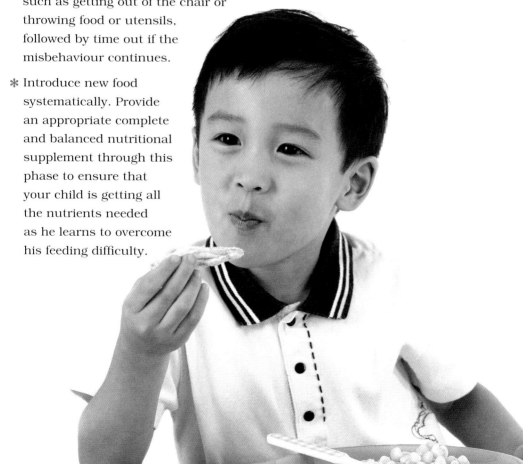

Obesity

Weight gain is a natural phenomenon that occurs in growing children, but many children today are at risk of gaining more weight than they should. Overweight children are prone to many health risks. Prevention is better than cure, so the best way to deal with excessive weight gain is to understand the causes and consequences and find out how you can protect your child from becoming obese.

Causes of Obesity

* Excessive food intake, especially high energy food choices. Children often load up on many additional calories from consuming sweetened drinks and snacks.

* Reduced physical activity. With high-rise living, children do not burn up as many calories as they should through active play. Television and computers have curbed activity even more. Unexpended energy just deposits fat in the body.

* Early nutrition. New insight suggests that excessive maternal weight gain during pregnancy results in large babies set for life with more fat cells than infants born within the normal range. Rapid weight gain in early life programmes the brain with a larger appetite and this increases an infant's risk of staying overweight. On the other hand, small babies that gain weight rapidly are also at greater risk of adult onset heart disease and diabetes.

Consequences of Obesity

* Childhood obesity adversely affects almost every organ system in the body.

* Excessive weight loads the bones and joints and these young children suffer constant pain.

* A host of risk factors such as high blood pressure, high blood cholesterol and diabetes set overweight children up for heart attacks and diabetes in adulthood.

* Many obese children suffer from breathing disorders.

Preventing Obesity

* The best place to start is always at the beginning, hence doctors advise expectant mothers to keep to an appropriate pregnancy weight gain. Starting life at the right weight helps each child have a fighting chance to stay trim and fit through life. Mothers with diabetes should ensure good blood glucose control to prevent their babies from growing too large in the womb.

* Breastfeed. Studies have shown that exclusively breastfed infants have appropriate weight gain.

* Provide a well-balanced diet. You are the gatekeeper of your child's food choices. Offer your child a wide variety of nutrient-dense food choices at meal- and snack times and guide him on the appropriate amount to eat. Do not force him to finish his food if he is already full. Avoid serving high fat and highly sweetened food to help your child develop a preference for more nutritious choices. Set a good example for your child to follow.

* Ensure regular physical activity. Control the amount of time your child spends each day on sedentary activities such as watching television, playing on the computer or with handheld games, studying or sitting quietly. Organise time for active play each day and encourage participation in sports and games. Play with your child and exercise regularly. Your child will take his cue from what you do rather than what you say.

Losing the Weight

Once a child has gained more weight than he should, it takes greater effort to help him lose it, but patience and perseverance will pay off.

* Help your child expend his energy by modifying his daily activities and encouraging more active play. For example, instead of watching television or playing computer or handheld games, encourage your child to play outdoors.

* Cutting back on food is not appropriate as children are still growing. Instead, offer your child healthier choices in his daily diet, such as fresh fruit instead of sweets and biscuits, and baked rather than fried dishes.

Bladder and Bowel Control

Generally, children gain control of the muscles that regulate the bladder and bowel when they are between 18 and 24 months old. Some children develop later. Toilet training should start only when your child is ready.

Toilet Training

Here are some signs to show that your toddler may be ready for toilet training.

* Stays dry for at least two hours at a time.

* Has bowel movements at particular times of the day.

* Asks to be changed out of a wet or soiled diaper.

* Can pull his pants down and up again.

* Is able to follow instructions.

Ready, Set, Go!

Introduce the Idea

When your toddler is ready, buy him a potty. Better still, take him to the shop with you and let him pick one that he likes. Talk about what the potty is for in simple terms. Let him sit on it from time to time, at first just for fun. You may want to dump the contents of a soiled diaper into the potty to show him what it is for. Let your toddler see family members of his sex use the toilet to clue him in.

Schedule Toilet Breaks

Have him sit on the potty with his diaper off first thing in the morning, after meals and before and after a nap. Praise him whenever he urinates or defecates in the potty.

Catch His Cues

As soon as you notice signs such as squatting, squirming or holding his genital area, make a beeline for the potty and tell him you want him to urinate and defecate in it.

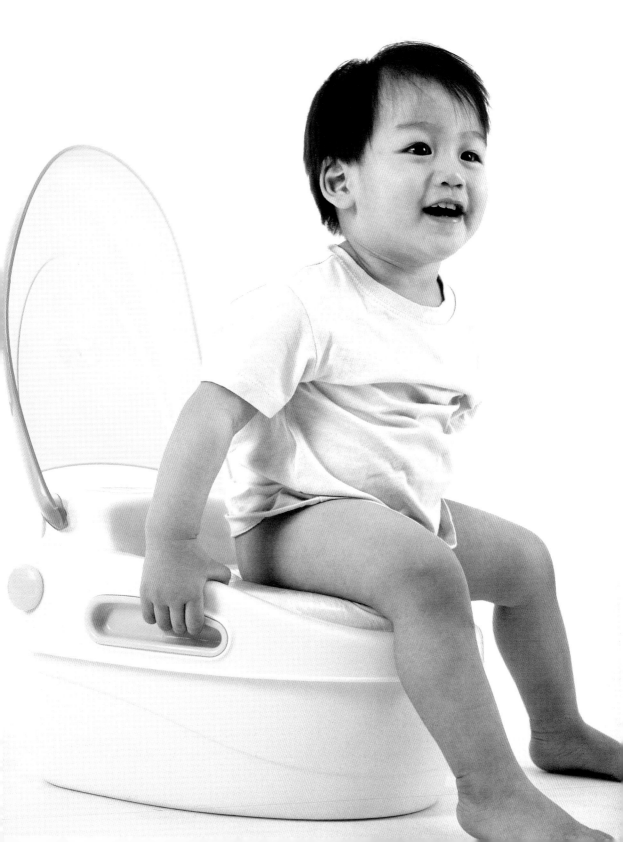

Give Incentives

Lavish him with praise and offer rewards like a trip to the park or extra bedtime stories for his successes. Be positive and do not scold or nag him for unsuccessful attempts.

Ditch the Diapers

After he has been using the potty successfully for a few days, let him move on to training pants or regular underwear. Celebrate the occasion by taking him on a 'big boy' outing. Have him hear you tell family members and friends about what a big boy he is.

Overlook Accidents

Do not punish or scold him when he wets or soils himself. This will happen for a while, especially when he is tired or upset.

Do Not Force It

If your toddler resists the potty or just isn't getting the hang of it, take a break. Chances are that he is not ready yet. Try again in another month or so.

Learning to Use the Toilet

Once your toddler is toilet trained, get him accustomed to using the toilet. Put a padded toilet training seat over the adult seat to make it more comfortable for him.

Sit with him to help him to develop confidence in using the toilet as some children have a fear of falling into it.

Flush the toilet only after he gets off the toilet seat as some children are frightened by the sound of the gushing water.

Bedwetting

Most children should be dry at night by the time they are about 5 years old. By the time they are 6 or 7 years old, only about 10 percent of them will continue to wet their beds at night.

Bedwetting is more common in boys than girls. And it may run in the family. If one parent had a history of bedwetting, there is a 50 percent chance of their child having the same problem. And the incidence goes up to 70 percent if both parents wet their beds when they were young.

Bedwetting is involuntary and the child has no control over wetting. Punishing or shaming your child will only cause emotional and behavioural problems. Factors causing bedwetting include:

* Hereditary causes.

* Deep sleep. Your child is unable to wake up to go to the toilet.

* Delay in maturation of the bladder. Without treatment, bedwetting decreases over time with only 1 percent of children continuing to bedwet after puberty.

* Lack of an anti-diuretic hormone that reduces urine production at night.

Without treatment, your child should stop bedwetting as he grows older. However, if you are concerned that he is still wetting himself at night, several times a week or every night, see your family doctor.

Bedwetting can be treated with drugs to reduce urine production at night and/or with the use of an alarm to gradually condition your child to wake up in the middle of the night to go to the toilet.

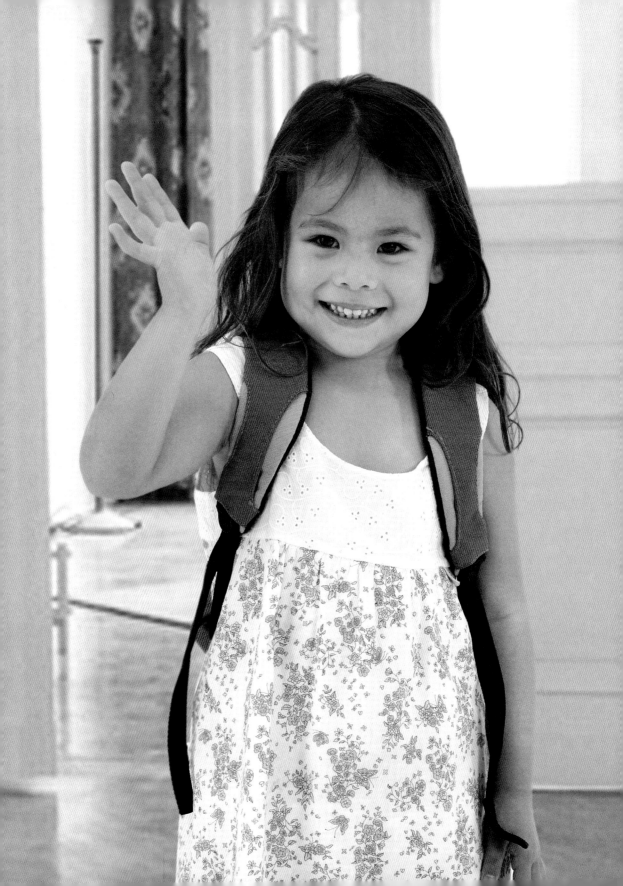

Your
Preschooler

Much as you want your child to be intelligent,
you also want him to grow up to be an all-rounded
person with strong emotional and social skills. Provide
your child with opportunities to develop language to
communicate and express his thoughts and feelings,
and ensure he has a secure home environment where
he knows that he is loved unconditionally.

Contributors:

Asst Prof Linda Gan
Mrs Kathleen Chia
Dr Pamela Sharpe

Pregnancy   0 to 1 month   2 to 11 months   12 months to 3 years   3 to 6 years

Speech, Reading and Writing Skills

Language Development

You play a major role in your child's language development. Apart from talking to your baby even before he can say actual words, you will find, in this chapter, activities that can help to develop your child's speech and expand his vocabulary.

How Language Develops

Speaking is an important milestone, possibly even more so than walking for many Asian parents. It is something parents talk about and compare, and lateness in developing speech causes anxiety.

Both speaking and walking develop at about the same time, with some children concentrating on one and some on the other. Early speech is not necessarily a sign of precociousness. Lateness in speaking, as in walking, can be genetic as well as related to gender.

Boys are often slower than girls in developing speech and walking, and various reasons have been suggested for this: notable differences in the wiring of the brain and carers, often women, speaking more to girls than to boys, with this perhaps influencing brain development.

Pattern and Sequence of Development in the Preschool Years

Age	Understanding and Speaking
3 to 4 years	Understands and responds to questions
	Uses correct word order in sentences most of the time
	Vocabulary expands rapidly
	Continues to have difficulty with some speech sounds
	In English: Uses regular verbs like "play" and "walk" correctly and may use regular plurals like "boys" (Plurals are often difficult for non-native speakers.)
	Experiments with grammar and may say things like "rided"
	Talks about what he is doing as he is doing it—the here and now
	Talks to himself as he plays
	Uses questions to ask "Why", "When" and "How"
4 to 6 years	Understands approximately 2,000 words and has a large vocabulary
	Understands time sequence
	Understands rhyming
	Articulates almost all speech sounds correctly
	Sentences are more complex and detailed
	Can tell a story using his imagination
	Describes people and objects and can engage in conversation
	Talks about kindergarten and home, about yesterday and the future
	May use language to shock adults

Girls Listen Better

Girls appear to be better listeners, even from young, so boys need plenty of practice: name the things your child points to; sing nursery songs and rhymes; name things in simple books while resisting the temptation to try and get the child to repeat after you!

Learning through Interaction

Although the development of language comes naturally—crying, cooing, babbling, first words—the opportunities to use language and the encouragement that your child receives will have a positive impact on his skills.

Children need face-to-face interaction in order to learn to talk: someone who cares to speak to and respond to them in a way they can understand. Even before a child can utter a word, most parents and carers instinctively recognise the language potential of their child and speak to him, and this is very important.

Learning through Listening

Before speaking, your child has spent a long time listening to and tuning into the language or languages he has heard around him. He will understand many words before he can start using them. This refers to the receptive language ability as opposed to expressive language ability. By his second year, your child will understand more and more words. At 3 years, he will begin to understand simple instructions and concepts. This is the time to build up his receptive vocabulary with lots of listening activities.

Grasping Language

In the beginning, your child may have difficulties with pronunciation and understanding. Those who are close to your child may understand his language, but others may not. This is a good reason for keeping carers constant or your child's desire to make himself understood can be frustrated.

Very sensibly, children simplify pronunciation before they master it, saying things like "poon" for spoon. Some examples of the sounds that children find difficult in English and tend to simplify are:

* *Sh* for "s", as in "yesh" for "yes"

* *D* for "th", as in "de" for "the". This sound remains difficult for Chinese speakers as does the "r" sound, which is replaced with "l"

* *F* for "th", as in "fin" for "thin"

* *V* for "th", as in "fever" for "feather"

* *W* for "r", as in "wase" for "race"

* *L* for "y", as in "lellow" for "yellow"

With correct modelling, difficulties in pronunciation usually disappear by the age of 5 or 6.

Baby Talk

Mispronunciation can appear cute and it is tempting to continue using such words with your child. However, this is not very helpful. Children need to hear the correct pronunciation, even if they cannot as yet make the correct sounds themselves.

Similarly, when your child starts speaking, you may find yourself still using baby talk—either copying your child or using baby words for things like milk, food, the pacifier, the toilet and parts of the body. It is not uncommon to hear things like "You want your mum-mum now?" While there is little harm in this, if you use the correct word, your child will not have to unlearn it later.

If you have been using baby talk with your child, use his birthday or other milestone to break the habit. You can say something like "Now you are 3, we are going to call your *weewee* your penis. That's the right word."

Motherese or Parentese

The way parents and carers adjust their language to help the child's understanding is referred to as "motherese" or "parentese". This does not mean that you have to resort to ungrammatical language. For example, you may offer your child a choice by saying "Milk or juice?" Later, the same choice can be phrased to "Do you want milk or juice?" with the important words, "milk" and "juice", emphasised. Imagine yourself trying to speak to someone who does not understand English—that is the way to help your child in his language development.

Learning the Rules of Language

Children make grammatical errors as they teach themselves the rules of a language and the exceptions. This means that if you want your child to speak a language well, you need to ensure that the adults around him speak that language well.

As children learn to talk, they love to hear the sound of their own voices, so try recording your child as he talks and sings. This is also a good way for you and your child to see what progress he has made as you play back what he was saying a few weeks ago and compare it to what he can manage at the present moment.

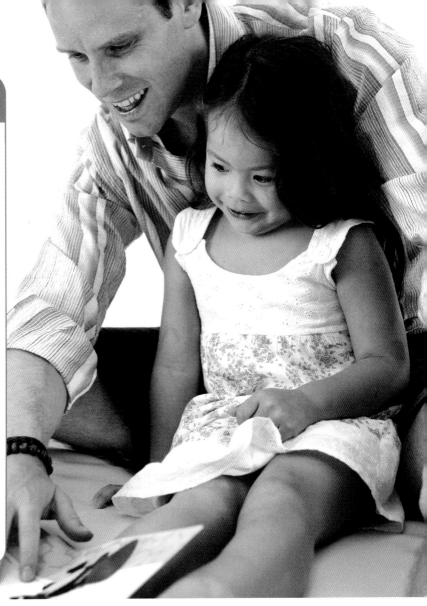

Spotting Problems

If you suspect your child has a hearing problem or is not reaching his milestones in language development, it is advisable to take him for a hearing assessment with an audiologist.

Hearing difficulties are the most common cause of language delay. Hearing is checked at birth but hearing loss may develop later as a result of infections and colds.

Inform your child's teachers of any hearing difficulties your child has so they can make allowances, like placing your child at the front of the group.

Some children have high tone deafness and cannot hear consonants properly. If you find that your child ignores a lot of what you say or frequently responds with "What?", he may have a hearing difficulty and not just selective hearing!

Speech Delay

Lateness in learning to talk can be the result of the child not getting enough individual attention from adults and from lack of encouragement. Boys need to be spoken to, especially in families where more talkative girls may dominate the talk that goes on.

Whenever you can, restrict distractions from background sounds like TV and other speakers, even another child, when talking to your child. Have your own special quiet time to talk. Children need the individual attention of a caring parent and the time to listen and talk in order to develop communication skills. You can read a book with him or teach him a rhyme or song.

DEVELOPING VOCABULARY

Pointing is an important gesture that aids vocabulary development. Children point not only to what they want, but often to what they want named. They begin processing these names which in time become a part of their vocabulary. A child needs to hear a word 500 to 600 times before he starts to use it himself so naming what the child is interested in or pointing to is very important.

Expanding and extending is a good way of helping your child to develop his vocabulary. For example:

> Toby : Bird!
>
> Adult : Oh yes! I can see the bird.
>
> Toby : Bird fly!
>
> Adult : Yes, the bird is flying. It's using its wings.

Another way is to use fill-ins:

> Adult : The bird is using its...
>
> Toby : Wings!

Children do not seem to respond to correction as they do not understand what the adult is trying to correct. Providing the correct model works better:

> Jason : I gotted new shoes.
>
> Adult : Yes, you have got a new pair of shoes.

Stammering

As your child's language develops, his thoughts may race ahead of his ability to express himself, and he may begin to stumble over or repeat words, as if stalling for time to get his thoughts in order. This is called "stuttering" or "stammering". It is usually a temporary phase that children pass through. Some encouragement like "Take your time. I'm listening", may be all your child needs. Do not assume a problem is developing unless the stammering persists. Fussing about it and showing impatience will increase your child's anxiety and not help the situation.

SIGNING

Well before your child can talk, he will use body language to make his needs known; wriggling when he wants to be put down; stretching out his hands when he wants to be picked up; pushing you towards something he wants; and of course using his eyes, head and other hand signals.

The signs and gestures your child uses are an imperfect form of communication. You may not be quite sure what your child wants when he points to the shelf—the book or the soft toy—but you will soon find out as the wrong item will be firmly rejected and thrown down!

Dr Linda Acredolo and Dr Susan Godwin co-authored a book called *Baby Signs*. Together with Joseph Garcia, an American scientist who worked with the deaf, they developed the *Sign with Your Baby* programme. Although they had intended the programme for babies 6 months and older, in Singapore, classes using this programme are offered to babies as young as 3 months old. The system is said to benefit children as old as 3 years, easing them into an enjoyment of literature by acting out the words in picture books with signs and actions. The programme looks like it is here to stay and has produced a mass of books, CDs, DVDs, kits, workshops and classes.

There is lots of information on the web about baby signing programmes with articles by professionals and parents who are both enthusiastically for and against it. Parents should check these out to make an informed decision before buying into any of these programmes.

SELF-TALK

You may notice that as your child engages in a task like trying to fit Lego blocks together, he talks about what he is doing. This self-talk is speech that is helping your child to think. As adults, we do this inside our heads. Your child will also do likewise as he matures.

You can help him to use language to think logically by talking about what you are doing with him such as going through a shopping list in the market or supermarket, making a cake, washing your car, buying and writing a birthday card and folding the washing, etc. Although it may be easier and quicker to do these things by yourself, these are wonderful learning opportunities if you involve your child and talk to him about what you are doing. Here is an example of talking through a task with a child:

Adult:

Let's find all the socks. Now we have to match them, like this. (You demonstrate finding pairs.)

Now Mummy will roll them together.
Look, two socks in one now!

Okay, now you put Papa's socks here and your socks there. Then we will go and put them in the drawers.

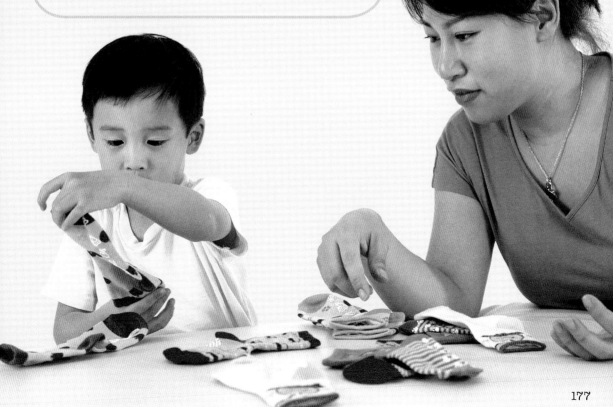

Multilingualism

Living with multiple languages is a common experience, especially in Asia. Languages provide a unique view of how particular cultures view the world. In Singapore, the view is that learning your mother tongue will help you preserve your cultural heritage and Asian values.

Multilingualism and Development

Research shows that children in bilingual families reach the same basic milestones and at the same rate as monolingual children. They start using words and begin producing sentences about the same time.

A Multilingual Environment

Having two or more world views from learning different languages has to be better than one. Indeed, the advantages of learning in a multilingual environment have been well researched and documented. These include:

* A heightened awareness of how language works.

* Flexibility of thinking, which helps with problem solving as the child is able to switch between languages.

* Greater sensitivity to others from a young age.

Managing Multilingualism

Will your child get confused when presented with two languages? And will it cause language delay?

The expert consensus is that the child will not, provided the languages are used one at a time or kept separate. The window of opportunity for learning an additional language is open until about 10 to 12 years of age, during which time children absorb and learn languages almost as if they are one big language.

What is important is that children attain some proficiency in the languages they speak. Using a bicycle analogy, having two languages, neither of which is really proficient, is like having a bike with two square wheels. It will take the child nowhere. Being proficient in two languages is like having a bike with two good wheels. It will take the child places. Even having a bike with one big wheel—or one proficient language—and another small wheel—some grasp of another language—will be more useful. This does not mean that the child will not mix languages. If he does not have the necessary word in one language but knows it in another, he will use that. In multiple language environments like Singapore, languages are 'mixed', with users discerning which word in Malay, Mandarin, dialect or English expresses its meaning best.

Be Consistent

There are various ways in which you can introduce language to your child. In Singapore, many households follow a pattern of simultaneous bilingualism, where two or more languages are introduced and acquired together before the child is 3 years old. Having a parent speak to the child consistently in a language and the other parent or carer in another language seems to work well, especially if they are good language models.

Be serious and committed to raising a bilingual child, but do not be so rigid that you cannot relax or relapse into the other language if the social situation requires it.

Make Language Learning Fun

Songs, rhymes and stories on tapes, CDs and DVDs can be useful for tuning your child in to the sounds of the language. Even if your child is reluctant to speak, keep at it and make it, if possible, a daily, positive experience. You can make it fun by learning it together with your child.

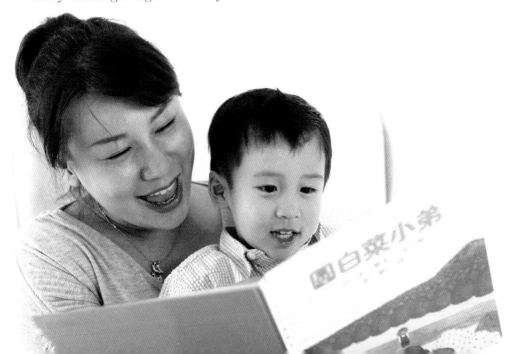

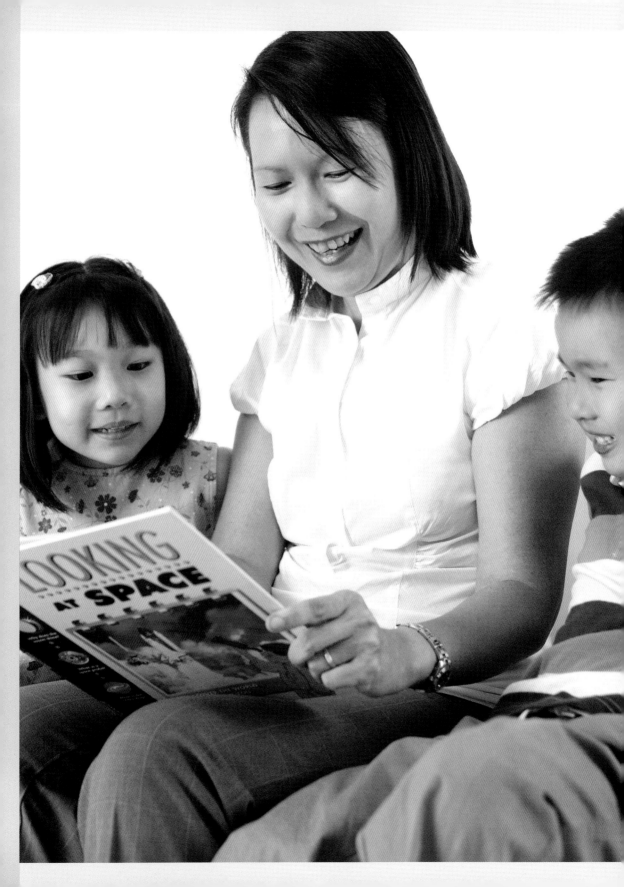

YOUR CHILD'S ENDLESS QUESTIONS

From the time he is about 2½ years old, your child will begin to ask questions. He will begin by asking "What" and "Who" type questions, progressing to "Where" around 3 years old and at 4 years, will be asking "When", "Why" and "How".

This progression mirrors your child's progress in thinking and understanding concepts of time, place, people and events past and present. While this can be exasperating for you at times, it is your child's way of finding out and making sense of his world. Your child will acquire and absorb a great deal of information if his observations are encouraged and his questions answered.

You may not always know the answers and it is all right to say you do not know and then take steps to find out. You will not lose face with your child if you admit that you are not a walking encyclopaedia.

If you are tired, say so. If you see the questions as a ploy to delay bedtime, be firm but not angry and nasty. Your child may crave your attention but he needs to know you have limits. Try throwing the question back to your child to promote his thinking, such as "Why do you think monkeys have long tails?"

Reading and Writing

Learning to read is not as natural a skill as learning to speak. The world is full of people who can speak but for whom reading and writing remain a challenge. Since both are important skills, introduce them in ways that will encourage your child to want to learn.

Reading

Reading involves two processes: being able to work out what words say (decoding skills) and being able to take meaning from them (understanding or comprehension). Both are important.

Your child may be able to read or decode words but may not know what they mean because they are not in his spoken vocabulary or part of his experience. If that is the case, reading will not be a satisfying, meaningful process. He may master it but not enjoy it and may never know the joy of curling up with a good book. This is why you should not hurry your child into being able to read. Having a good vocabulary is an important prerequisite for reading.

Letter Names and Sounds

Once your child starts noticing letters, invest in a set of magnetic letters that can be displayed on the fridge. Have fun using them to form his name and the names of other family members or important words for him.

Find a set of letters that has the vowels and consonants in two different colours—or paint them yourself—this will introduce your child to the two types of letters needed to make words. The process of learning to read will take off from there.

Start by teaching your child the letter sounds, for example the sound for "B" should be as in the beginning of the word "ball" and not "bee". He will be able to use the letter sounds that he has learnt to read words.

When making words with magnetic letters, try to use the letter sounds and only use capital letters where appropriate.

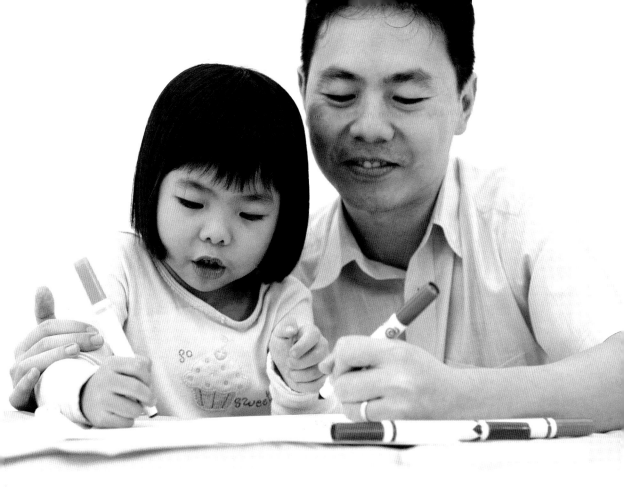

Once children begin wanting to write the letters, teach lower case and capitals together. Capitals are easier to form but children are not going to meet them in print as much as lower case letters.

Writing

Writing begins with making marks on paper. When children see adults writing, they want to do it too. At first, it will look like scribble but it may well have meaning for your child. You can ask your child to tell you what his 'writing' says. As your child becomes more interested in letters, you can begin to write something of what he has said to you at the bottom of his 'writing', explaining that it is just so you don't forget his story. Soon, you will begin to see letters of the alphabet appear in his writing and you will know that the process of writing is beginning.

Letters of the Alphabet

Even among Singaporean adults, it is common to confuse letters for alphabets which they are not. The English alphabet consists of 26 letters, A to Z.

Reading to Your Child

Reading a book with your child can be a very special time of intimacy and bonding. It also communicates to your child that reading is important and can help lay the foundation for a lifelong love for reading in him.

Lap Reading

Make an early start with lap reading—when your child is small enough to sit on your lap—and before he begins moving around so that he will associate books with sitting, looking and listening, and participating by turning the pages and imitating sounds.

Benefits of Reading to Your Child

The Beginning of Literacy

All research suggests that children who are read to are being given the best start in learning to be literate. It really is as simple as that—read to your child. Researchers have found that "children who are read to every day at three are likely to be flourishing in a wide range of subjects by the age of five", so there is truth in the old adage:

> *You may have tangible wealth untold;*
> *Caskets of jewels and coffers of gold.*
> *Richer than I you can never be—*
> *I had a mother who read to me.*
> ~Stricklan Gilligan (1869–1954)

A Love for Books

Reading to your child can be the beginning of a lifelong enjoyment of books and reading, as your child starts to associate reading with pleasure and emotional satisfaction, and is motivated to try to read himself.

Develop Vocabulary, Increase Knowledge and Engage Imagination

The experience of reading with you can lead your child to develop a fascination for words, their sounds and meanings and hence stretch his vocabulary.

When you read different genres or types of material—stories, rhymes, poems, folk tales, information books—to him, you introduce him to written language that will help him expand his knowledge and horizons and engage his imagination. It also makes him aware of book language—"Once upon a time", "A long time ago... lived happily ever

184

after", "The end"—that he can imitate in his own story telling and later in his story writing. The list of benefits goes on.

Reading Comprehension

Helping your child to understand what he sees and hears when you are reading to him is important because it prepares him for a successful start at school.

Start with books that have one or two objects to a page, talk about each object, relating it to his experience, and ask questions about it. In this way, your child learns to listen, focus attention and give responses. As he moves to storybooks, engage him in discussion around the story by asking such questions as "What part did you like best?", "What would you do if you were the crocodile?" and "Do you think that was a good thing to do?"

This encourages your child to think, give his opinions and use his imagination and creativity. These are more sophisticated or higher order skills that are important in further developing reading comprehension and writing skills.

Another good thing about storybooks is that they can lead from talking about the story to chatting about everyday life. If you find it difficult to talk to your child, use stories to get you started.

Let Your Child Lead

Try to curb your enthusiasm to teach and let your child take the lead in pointing out letters or words. Sessions should be kept short and enjoyable. Let your child ask for more but be alert to this being a delay tactic, especially at bedtime.

Share Stories

Your child will love to hear stories about himself as a baby and about the things you did as a child—these are a part of his personal history and family heritage. Together with cuddles, these are also times for telling your child how much you love him. Your child needs to hear this and experience your touch every day in order to develop well emotionally and socially.

The Same Story Over and Over!

Does your child enjoy having the same story read over and over to him? While it may be boring for you, he is in fact concentrating on different elements of the story during these times and confirming his knowledge of it. Try skipping a few pages and you will know this is true!

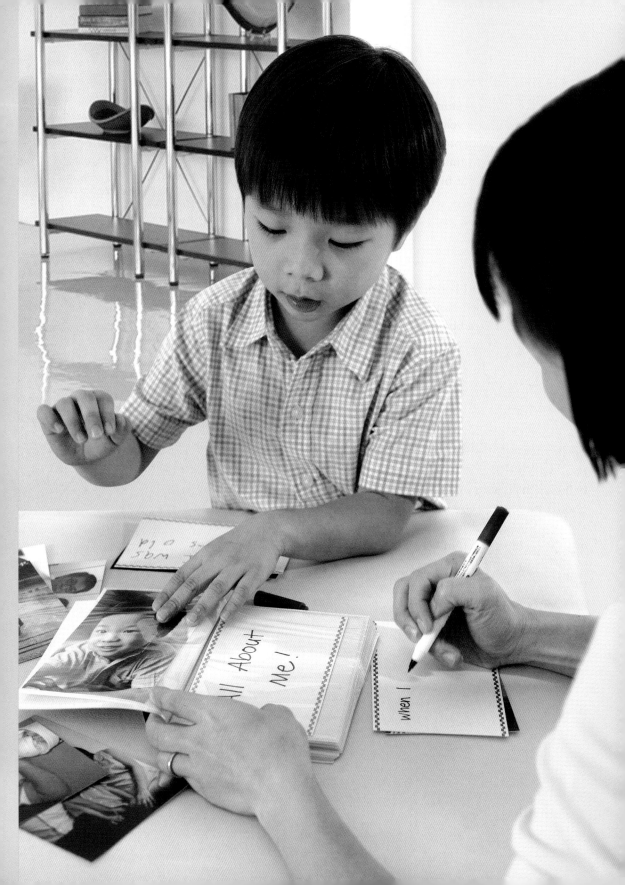

Listen to Rhymes, Stories and Songs

Listening to rhymes, stories and songs are other wonderful ways of helping to develop your child's language and stimulating his imagination. These can be provided by CDs, DVDs and TV programmes but be there to interact with your child about what he sees and hears.

Encourage Variety, Allow for Favourites

Libraries are well stocked with children's books. Your child may discover new interests or deepen his existing ones through the different books on offer.

Second-hand book stores, sales and other families are also good sources of books. It is a good idea to go for variety but allow for favourites. Do not choose only alphabet books, having teaching in mind, or books about characters that your child has seen on TV programmes or in computer games.

Make Your Own Books

You can also make your own books about the family or holidays filled with photos and happy memories. The little photo albums that are available from photo developing shops are just right for small hands. Slot in some photos of your child involved in activities or of your child and significant people in the family. You can slip in captions such as "I am playing ball", "I am swimming", "I love Mummy", "I love Daddy" etc. These then become a first reading book.

Make Books Easily Accessible

Encourage your child to read by making books easily accessible to him. Place his favourite books on low shelves or in baskets where he can pick them up on his own whenever he feels like reading.

Your Child's Developing Mind

Learning starts before your child goes to school. In fact, from the time your child is born, he is learning every day. Cognitive development refers to your child's ability to think, learn and solve problems, and it is largely in your hands to help him develop his cognitive abilities or thinking skills.

How Your Child Thinks

From the age of about 12 weeks, for example, your child is already aware of the abstract notion of cause and effect. He will discover that when he cries, he will attract attention and comfort from you or his caregiver. At a more sophisticated level, your child will come to learn about cause and effect relating to things in his immediate environment. For example, by pressing one of the buttons on the TV set or TV remote control, images will appear. In time, he will be able to sort things, classify them, then store and retrieve them from his memory. The ability to do these things is an important step towards the development of your child's thinking skills.

Your child is driven to make sense of his world in the same way he is driven to walk and talk. He is typically full of energy, dashing to and fro, rushing into things without a moment's hesitation, regardless of the danger he might be in! He will ask endless questions and demand attention from those around him about whatever is intriguing him at the time.

How You Can Help

You can help your child extend his thinking skills by providing opportunities with simple everyday objects for him to match and sort by shape, size, colour and patterns, for example. In the process, your child will develop his ability to remember and recall the new information learnt. Toys like puzzles, matching games and construction toys also develop these abilities.

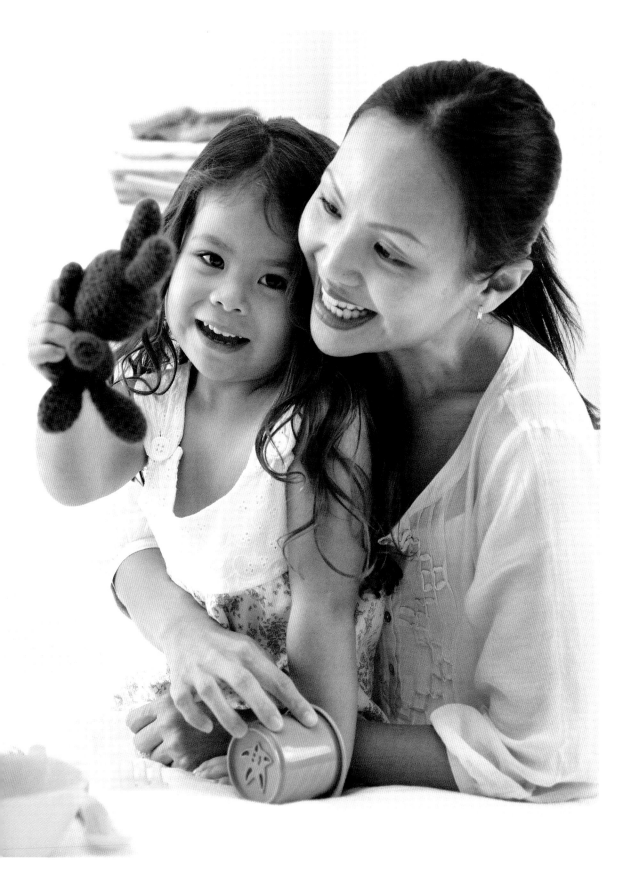

Age	Milestones for Cognitive Development
3 to 4 years	Distinguishes between heavy and light, long and short
	Matches an object to another, for example chopsticks to bowls
	Sorts simple things into groups, for example toys and items of clothing
	Recognises and names the primary colours—blue, red and green
	Names three shapes
	Retells a simple story
	Counts 10 objects with an adult's help
4 to 5 years	Gives you a specific number of objects when asked, for example "Give me two blocks"
	Names five textures
	Names times of the day related to routine activities, for example breakfast and bedtime
	Recognises and names eight colours
	Matches symbols (numbers and letters)
	Selects heavy/light objects
	Acts on simple prepositions, for example "behind", "beside" and "next to"
	Rote counts up to 20
	Uses a simple map to navigate a route
5 to 6 years	Accurately counts up to 20
	Writes own name
	Arranges objects according to size
	Names and orders the days of the week
	Tells you the date/day of birthday
	Reads 10 or more words on sight
	Tells you what might happen next, for example in a story
	Shows you half and whole objects, for example half a bar of chocolate
	Rote counts up to 100
	Understands that map symbols refer to real world objects

Adapted from: Tassoni P. & Beith K. *Child Care and Education*, page 201

DEVELOPING MEMORY

Children in preschool are in the process of developing their memories. Here are some tips on how you can sharpen your child's memory skills.

☐ Instead of nagging your child to remind him of everyday routines, post pictures up in relevant places. For example, put "Clean your teeth" on the bathroom mirror and "Take your school bag" on the front door.

☐ Get him to recall sequences of events. For example, ask him "What did you/we do yesterday?", "What are you/we going to do today?", "Do you remember where Daddy said we are going this Sunday?"

☐ Play memory games. Arrange several items on a tray. Give your child a few minutes to take a look at them, then cover the tray with a cloth and ask him to recall the items. If necessary, prompt him along with clues such as "There was a yellow fruit. What was it?"

Your Child's Memory

As toddlers become more competent at remembering their past and present experiences, they will be better able to organise their thinking and use their memory to help them plan for new situations. They will be able to think before they do instead of just rushing into things!

The Thinking Process

Your child does not learn effectively by being a passive observer. Just like a scientist, he needs to be actively involved in experimenting with everything around him and exploring different ideas in order to come up with his own theories.

Treasure Boxes

Make up treasure boxes with safe, natural objects from around the house with different textures for your young child to explore. For example, a silk scarf, a flannel, a sponge, a plastic bottle with a screw top and a toothbrush. Encourage him to ask you questions about these things. Record or take photographs of him investigating these objects for "Talk About" sessions with you later.

Young Scientist at Work!

Your young scientist needs time, space and patience on your part to test out his theories. Shopping centres, departmental stores, mealtimes, his play area, the living room and the bath, for example, will be his laboratories. Chaos is the natural order of the day as your child fiddles with his food, takes things apart, throws things around and becomes obsessive about repeating things over and over again in the process of confirming his hypotheses!

Amidst all this apparent chaos, however, your child is constantly learning new things. By building on his previous experience, he is developing general notions or ideas (called concepts) which he will use to solve problems and expand his learning.

Destroyer or Investigator?

Have you seen your child painstakingly build a tower of blocks for example and then destroy it? Your child is investigating everything in his immediate environment, even if it means dissecting things to see how they work. This is his way of refining key concepts which form the foundation for further learning, such as big and small, heavy and light.

Overlook the Mess

The progress young children make in being able to gradually reason things out by testing their different theories through hands-on experiments is remarkable. Do not pass up on the golden opportunity to further your child's thinking skills by constantly curtailing his efforts by scolding him for making a mess at home.

Bath time, for example, is an excellent time for your child to splash around in water and test the laws of physics! Your child is already acquainted with the laws of gravity, having dropped endless objects on the floor and knowing that these objects promptly fall to the ground. But in the bath, this theory is challenged.

Give him a variety of containers of different shapes and sizes, such as shampoo bottles and plastic food boxes. Let him experiment by filling the containers with water and then pouring it away. This will eventually lead him to conclude that bigger containers will take longer to empty because of the volume of water they are able to hold. He will also discover that water has different properties to air and that full containers behave differently from empty ones. When he tries to push an empty container down in the water to the bottom of the bath, he will discover that he has to exert a lot of force to do so and that he has to hold it there or it will bob up to the surface again!

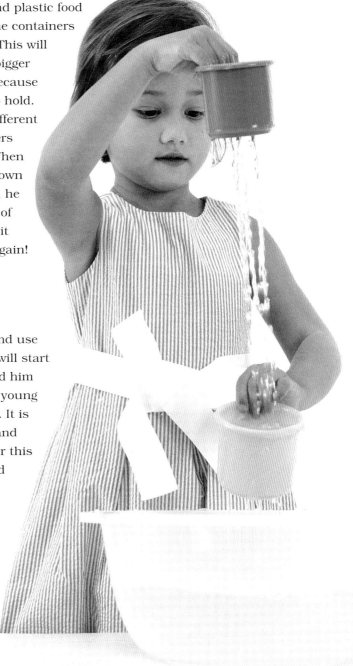

Talk to Your Child to Expand His Thinking

As soon as your child is able to talk and use language to express his thoughts, he will start to bombard you and the adults around him with questions. It is the principal tool young children have to extend their learning. It is therefore crucially important for you and the other adults around him to answer this torrent of questions in order to expand your child's thinking skills and his general knowledge.

You can generally expect your 2- to 3-year-old to ask "What" and "Who" questions and your 3- to 4-year-old to ask "Where", "When", "Why" and "How" questions.

Problem Solving

The drive to experiment will persist as your child progresses from 3 to 6 years. His memory improves day by day, enabling him to recall previous experiences and link different ideas to help him solve problems more effectively.

His skill in linking different ideas to follow a more logical system of thinking is evidenced in his more advanced ability to sort objects into their correct categories, or what appears to be his enthusiasm to tidy up! For example, he may start putting his storybooks on one shelf and his toys on another. This is a crucial step towards a more mature, adult way of thinking. By gradually reducing his environment to more manageable and comprehensible categories, your child is imposing greater order in his life and making his world a more comprehensible and less frustrating place.

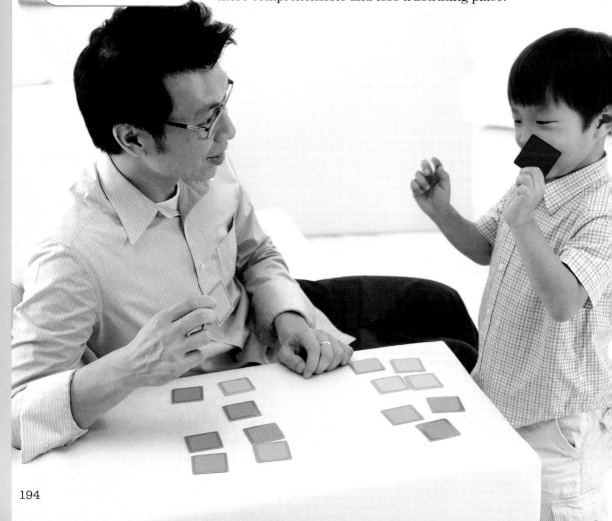

Challenge Thinking

It is important for you to continue providing varied opportunities to further challenge your child's thinking and the necessary equipment to help him test out his wrong hypotheses as well as his correct ones.

Guide your child in understanding why something happens, why it went right or wrong and what he can do the next time to produce a different outcome. Just telling him what will happen and the reasons why and leaving him to be a passive bystander in the process will deprive him of the critical experiences he needs to nourish his thinking skills.

Nurture Creative Thinking

Besides his scientific thinking, it is also important that you nurture your child's creative thinking. Creative thinking starts from watching and copying the actions of adults, for example picking up the telephone and pretending to speak after observing you doing so. Such imitation might seem unimportant and mundane but it is the first step your child is taking to use his imagination. Observe how your child, aided by an increasing level of sophistication in language skills, moves on to improvising and then creating his own telephone conversations. When you accompany your child in these imaginary events, however, resist imposing your own script for your child to follow. Simply listen and react but do not intrude on the experience your child is creating for you to participate in.

Allow Room to Grow

Resist the temptation to solve every single problem for your child. If your child is deprived of the opportunities to remember and/or strategise and innovate to overcome problems, his promotion to a more mature and flexible way of thinking may be delayed. Be patient and avoid hurrying your child to meet new intellectual challenges.

Counting from 10 to 20 in English is difficult as the teen numbers are irregular unlike other languages your child may be exposed to, such as Malay or Chinese. An example of difficult teen numbers include 11, 12 and 15.

CREATIVE WAYS TO TEACH BASIC CONCEPTS

Here are some activities you can use to help your child develop his understanding of some basic concepts.

Number	: Matching bowls with chopsticks
Opposites	: Going up and down the slide in the playground
Temperature	: Watching ice cubes melt in a glass
Time	: Counting down the days to his birthday
Length	: Comparing the length of two different drinking straws
Height	: Standing next to your child and pointing out the difference in height
Speed	: Rolling a toy car down a slope and then along a level surface
Size	: Sorting out objects according to size
Shape	: Sorting out objects according to shape
Pattern	: Drawing repeated patterns in the sand at the playground or beach
Volume	: Trying to fit a beach ball into two bags of different sizes
Capacity	: Pouring water into containers of different sizes
Mass	: Filling buckets with sand

COUNT WITH ME

Numbers, like letters of the alphabet, are symbols that your young child will become increasingly aware of from the time he is about 2½ years old.

He hears numbers being spoken—birthdays, telephone numbers, bus numbers, house numbers and numbers in nursery rhymes. Some of these numbers are just labels, such as in bus and house numbers, and others show quantities.

Start by counting things around you such as body parts, biscuits, sweets, steps and lift floors. As your child begins to grasp numbers, move on from cardinal numbers (numbers that denote quantity) to ordinal numbers (numbers that indicate position).

To teach ordinal numbers, talk about queues and arrange toys and things in order to help your child understand position words like *first*, *second* and *last*.

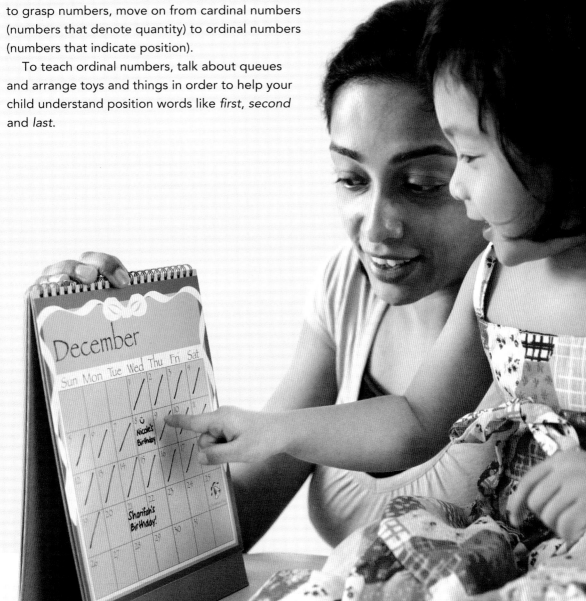

Accelerated Learning

Advertisements for early instructional programmes promise to advance children's thinking using innovative "brain training approaches". Many such advertisements claim, for example, to help children reach their milestones earlier and have longer attention spans. This has prompted many parents, aptly aided by educational entrepreneurs, to try and fast forward their children's cognitive growth through enrichment programmes.

True or False?

The evidence from brain research has generally been distorted by those who use this notion of "child competence" to justify engaging their young children in programmes aimed at advancing their intellectual capacity and learning ability. Below are just two of the myths that have arisen.

Myth One Use Them or Lose Them

Finding : Babies are born with an excess of brain cell connectors (called synapses).

Myth : If these connections are not used, they are lost forever!

Neuroscientists have found that before birth and in early childhood, children are born with an abundance of brain cells (or neurons) that are responsible for sending messages around the brain and from the brain to the body. Synapses connect brain cells and develop very quickly, especially in infants. For example, a 1-year-old child has 150 percent more synapses than an adult. Scientists suggest this overproduction possibly enables the neurons in the brain to respond sensitively to the demands of the child's environment. As part of normal, healthy development, nature prunes the unused synapses. Many people misunderstand this pruning process and fear that if these connections are not used, they are lost forever. This is not the case. The brain cells remain intact for later learning.

Myth Two All Critical Learning Takes Place Before 3 Years

Finding : The brain has growth spurts during the first three years of life. These years are of critical importance for laying the foundations for future learning.

Myth : After 3 years old, the windows of opportunity for young children to learn are closed.

Neurological research has helped us understand that there are optimal or best times for children to learn and that the brain can be likened to a sponge mopping up knowledge at an incredible rate during the first three years of life. This finding, however, has been misinterpreted by many parents who start their babies or toddlers on programmes at home or outside in the hope that they can accelerate their learning, such as flashing word cards at 6-month-old babies who have not yet learnt to talk in order to advance their reading skills.

Take Note

- Do not confuse formal learning with learning through play, from which very young children can learn an enormous amount.
- Extra stimulation over and beyond active interaction with sensitive and supportive parents will not necessarily build a genius child.

Evaluate Programmes Carefully

With the current focus on helping children realise talent other than academic skills, there is an even greater risk of children as young as 2 years old being exposed to brain enrichment programmes, and 3-year-olds to other courses such as art, music, logic or physical fitness to boost their chances of later success at school.

Take Note

- Evaluate these programmes carefully to decide whether your child will benefit from them.
- Sit in on a session before signing up.
  (I remember a drama class I wanted my son to join which just involved singing nursery rhymes and colouring worksheets. Needless to say, I did not enrol him.)

Proceed with Caution

Early childhood research suggests that parents should proceed with caution when trying to push their children ahead of the optimal times of development as their children run the risk of:

- Burning out by the ages of 8 and 9 years.
- Being put off school (which might well be teaching them things they have already been introduced to).
- Being thrown into emotional turmoil if they cannot meet the expectations that their parents have set for them. This can result in low self-esteem.
- Becoming unpopular social misfits, which impedes their efforts to develop the necessary social skills for meaningful interaction with others in life.

The Importance of Play

According to early childhood educators, it is important for parents to allow their children to enjoy childhood with adequate time set aside for them to play. They need to pursue their own ideas, discover and explore in a stress-free environment. This process should not be eroded by enrolling them in a string of structured learning programmes. This will tend to make them become overdependent on parents providing activities for them. Such children are deprived of the opportunity to think and plan for themselves and are more likely to become easily bored.

Children and Play

It is natural and healthy for children to play, and having a child who does not play is a cause for concern. Nevertheless, many Asian parents find it hard to appreciate the value of play. Adults often use phrases like "They're only playing", "Stop playing about", and "Do your work now, you can play later". These statements indicate that play is perceived as something trivial.

Think back to your childhood when you played throwing and aiming games with marbles and stones; chasing games like police and thief, and hide-and-seek; spinning tops and hopscotch; and *masak masak* (cooking) with improvised materials. Although you did not know it then, these games provided opportunities for developing intellectual, physical, creative and social-emotional skills as well as other life skills.

Today, however, play is mostly linked to toys, and unless children are organised, parents feel that playing is a waste of valuable time. Part of the difficulty may also be that there is very often nothing to show at the end of playing, and parents want to see something tangible.

A Right to Play

There is no doubt that children enjoy playing and the fun aspect is one of its characteristics. Play is actually a child's right. All young mammals play, and it is not only enjoyable but also essential practice for life. People who have had a great influence on educational programmes place a high value on play. Maria Montessori asserted that "play is the child's work" while the great Russian psychologist Lev Vygotsky saw play as "the leading source of development in the preschool years".

Preschool Programmes Based on Play

Presently, many educational programmes at preschool level are based on play. In such play-based programmes, the emphasis is on self-directed learning rather than teaching. Your child is motivated to play and, through play, can develop positive attitudes to learning, like curiosity and persistence. Allowing your child time to play leads to learning and development in all areas—social, physical, intellectual, creative and emotional.

Social Development

On the social level, your child will learn to cooperate, negotiate, share, take turns and appreciate another child's point of view when playing together. Interacting with other children provides opportunities for your child to understand the feelings of others and will help him develop empathy.

Physical Development

The physical benefits of play are obvious: for practising and fine-tuning gross and fine motor skills. Physical activity plays a critical role in the creation of nerve-cell networks essential to learning. Some children are kinaesthetic learners and learn best by doing and moving. Running around and letting off steam can also help children concentrate and improve appetite and overall health.

Intellectual Development

All forms of play at preschool level involve the intellect or thinking, whether it is practice play as in riding a bicycle, pretend play like acting out roles in the home, construction play with equipment like building blocks or playing games with rules as in football and rounders, snakes and ladders or four-in-a-row.

Your child will develop a basic understanding of what materials can do through sand and water play, and blocks and construction sets will help him make sense of mathematical and scientific learning later on. He will develop confidence in using language particularly through pretend play as this involves planning and negotiating problems and roles.

Children with experience in pretend play have been found to be better at using and interpreting letters and numbers, as well as problem solving.

Creative Development

It is believed that the critical period for the development of creativity is between 3 and 5 years old. Help your child develop his creative thinking with games and activities that involve imagination, making choices and being flexible in his thinking.

Emotional Development

Play is a stress reliever and allows your child to develop empathy and caring behaviour. Pretend and fantasy play allow your child to address his own feelings, anxieties and fears, and understand, control and master them.

Types of Play

There are many types of play. As your child develops, he moves through different stages of play, gradually becoming more social.

Physical Play

Physical play involves children actively moving around playing ball, balancing, climbing, jumping and so on. Another form of physical play is rough and tumble play. Fathers often engage in this type of play and many children find it great fun. While it is often a father and son activity, girls can enjoy it too. Recent research shows that this type of play leads to greater social competence in adolescence if the father is sensitive and does not over-extend the child. Play fighting in boys is common from 3 years of age to adolescence.

Discovery or Exploratory Play

Discovery or exploratory play—finding out what a toy or object can do, as well as its size, shape, texture and colour— is a common form of play from infancy through childhood. Your child may also discover that toys can be broken and this creates the opportunity for you to teach him to take care of his possessions.

Language Play

Nursery-aged children use language to play, like greeting each other with silly names like "Hello, Mr Monkey", "Hello, Mr Crocodile", and they find this very entertaining. Throughout childhood, children make up rhymes and jingles that form a feature of their games.

Your child's natural interest in word play and repetition should be encouraged through nursery rhymes and songs. This is a fun way of introducing language to your child.

Manipulative or Construction Play

Manipulative or construction play involves the hands, eyes and brain working together and is good for developing coordination. Toys for this type of play include lacing toys, stacking toys, sorting toys and pounding toys. Your child will become more skilled with age and practice, and will learn more about cause and effect through this type of play.

Imaginative or Pretend Play

In imaginative or pretend play, children take on roles. Initially, these are those of the mummy, the daddy or the baby, but as a child's knowledge and experience of the world develops, these extend to the shopkeeper, the customer, the patient, the doctor, the dentist and others.

For this type of play, language is important. It begins around 12 to

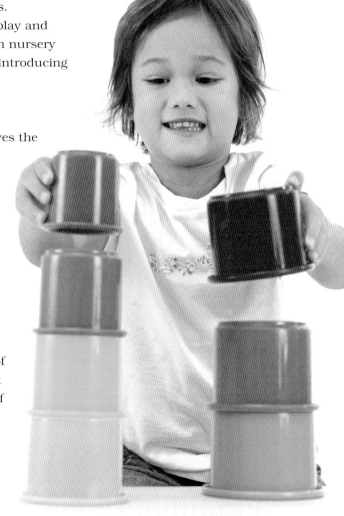

Some children develop an imaginary friend or companion. This usually happens between the ages of 3 and 9.

Studies suggest that far from being a cause for concern to parents, it exerts a positive influence on development with these children being highly socially interactive and more creative.

15 months and continues to 6 or 8 years. In this type of play, children frequently imitate the ways of adults. Pretending to be like someone else helps the child to understand other people's feelings and behaviour. Children choose different roles in fantasy play: girls tend to choose domestic roles while boys choose more masculine and active roles from TV or stories. However, boys should have the freedom to play house with dolls and girls should be able to take on what are seen as more masculine roles.

Creative Play

Creative play allows your child to express his feelings and ideas by making something out of clay or blocks, or through drawing and painting. Children can often express themselves more easily through these activities than through words, and this is the thinking behind using play or art as therapy.

Playing Games

Play that involves games with rules develops around the age of 6 to 7, with children playing more card and board games as well as games like hopscotch, chasing games and football. Children have to agree on the rules of these games and to any modifications. The transition from play to games is a gradual one and children need to be able to grasp that the rules need to be followed and that there is a reason for them. With time, your child will come to accept losing without floods of tears or a tantrum. It is best to avoid too much emphasis on competition until you see signs of this taking place.

Developing Social Skills

Socially, your child moves through different play stages gradually becomes more sociable and cooperative in play.

As a preschooler, your child should be able to play alone, play next to or with another child and play in a cooperative group. Sharing takes time and the inability to share is not a sign that your child is selfish but just that he is in the developmental stage of being self-centred. Having the experience of playing with others should lead to more cooperative play.

Through playing together with other children, your child will learn to negotiate and solve disagreements, provided you are not too quick to jump in and solve them for him. Children are far less likely than adults to give in, so children learn how other children react and how to manage conflicts.

Playing with others also teaches your child that anti-social behaviour like cheating and lying is not a way to keep friends. These are important skills and lessons in getting along with others that will apply throughout life.

Developing Concentration

Some children get really absorbed in play, others seem to flit from one thing to another. Having an adult's attention has been found to help children concentrate longer.

Try playing alongside your child. Use the same materials but do not take over the game or make the game too difficult. Your company will also help comfort and encourage your child.

Watching your child and making observant comments such as "I see you're trying to catch the bubbles with your hand" has also been found to be effective in helping children develop concentration.

Toys for Children

Children love visiting toy shops and they are good places to take your child to see what interests him. You can set the agenda before you go, such as telling your child, "This visit is just to look at the toys so we can think about what to buy for your birthday."

You have made a good choice if the toy is one your child really likes and uses often. It is pointless buying a toy or even a book that does not interest your child. Simple materials like cardboard boxes can make interesting toys for children to play with, becoming a cave, hidey-hole or even a boat!

Some Toys Are Necessary

Children need some toys. Toys give them pleasure and can make their games more varied and interesting. A good toy should be right for the age of your child (many toys have an age guide on the wrapping). It should be something that appeals to your child and leads him to take more than a fleeting interest in it, perhaps giving scope for thinking, imagination or learning new skills.

Not all toys have to be bought. They can be handed down from family to family or between friends' families, borrowed from friends, sourced from second-hand shops, the Internet and borrowed from toy libraries. Borrowing allows you to gauge how much a toy interests the child before deciding to buy it. Too much choice can be overwhelming for a child so a good tip is to put away toys that a child used to play with but appears to have lost interest in. Often the child's interest returns when the toy reappears a few weeks later.

Safe and Reliable Toys

Many countries producing toys have safety standards that follow approximately the model of the European Union Safety Standard. Marks to look for are:

* Lion mark. It is used by major international and European companies as a symbol of safety and quality.

* Kite mark. This means that the toy has been independently tested by the British Standards Institution, conforms to the relevant British Standard and should be safe and reliable.

* CE mark. Unlike the Lion and Kite marks, this symbol is not a European safety marker or quality symbol. It simply indicates that the toy has passed all European standards but may not necessarily have been tested for safety.

How to Choose a Toy

Ask yourself these questions when choosing a toy for your child.

* Is it sturdy and safe to play with?

* Does it have sharp edges and excessively small parts that may not be suitable for your child's age?

* Does it require a great deal of adult help to use it?

* Does it use a lot of batteries and/or require maintenance?

* Can you stand the noise it makes?

* Is it a mechanical or battery-operated toy that works at the push of a button? If so, will the novelty of the toy wear off quickly and will your child soon become bored and restless? Such toys are often easily broken and may lead to carelessness and destructiveness on the part of the child.

* Do you have sufficient storage space for the toy at home?

Top Toys

Top toys are toys that have a lasting interest for children. Such toys will engage your child's imagination and draw upon his creativity for months and even years to come. Examples of such top toys include:

* A good set of blocks.

* Dolls and soft toys. These can be very popular with some children but not interest others at all, so be guided by your own child. Simple dolls and soft toys allow scope for the imagination. Many children have a favourite doll, teddy or soft toy that is important to them for companionship and comfort throughout childhood.

* Books that allow younger children to use their imagination and older children to read for themselves.

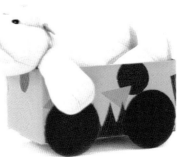

* Drawing and painting materials.

* Construction toys with mini people.

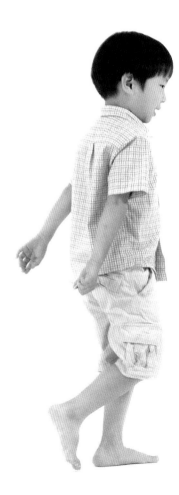

* Programmable toys like Roamers (educational robots that can be used for maths and language activities).

* Remote control cars.

* Dressing up outfits.

* Balls, tricycles, cars and bicycles for active play.

* Puzzles for developing concentration.

* Computer games and kits for making things for children 5 years and above.

Banning Toys

Many parents worry about toys like swords and guns that may lead to violent play, particularly amongst boys. Research has shown that children learn aggressive attitudes and behaviour more from viewing violence in the media than from the toys, so limiting your child's exposure to violence may have a greater effect than banning toys.

Most preschools have a policy of not allowing such toys, but if you prohibit them at home as well, your child will often find other things to use and improvise with. It can be a tricky situation as once your child realises it is something you disapprove of, it may become even more exciting for him. Some children may also think they can do the feats of Superman or Spiderman, confusing fantasy with reality, so rather than doing away with toys, talk to your child about the difference between fantasy and reality, and emphasise kindness and not hurting others when he engages in play fights with his friends.

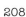

PLAYING TOGETHER

Your child needs to play by himself, with other children and sometimes with an adult. The tendency is to ignore your child when you think he is happily playing but sometimes sitting down and noticing what he is doing, referred to as play listening, is something your child will appreciate and is good for his self-esteem. Provide a commentary rather than asking questions. You may say something like "Oh, I see you are using lots of blue in your picture. Now you are using red." This allows the child to open up and tell you more about what he is doing and even enlist your help if he wants to.

Set aside time for just having fun together. You can take your child to a nearby park to play frisbee or ball or fly a kite. You can even wash the family car together—the important thing is to give your child your undivided attention. Such moments will make up an important part of your child's memories when he grows up.

Where parents choose to get involved with their children at or out of the home, perhaps volunteering at their school, there are always costs in terms of time but the benefits for the child are priceless. Research shows that children perform better at school when parents are involved.

Social and Emotional Development

Development of Self

You play an important role in helping your child grow up with a healthy, stable and balanced view of himself. With your love and support, you can help your child become socially and emotionally competent, providing him with a secure foundation for future growth and development.

Constructing Self Concepts

The exciting but complex process of building a picture of who we are and constructing our sense of self begins during the first year of life and continues to develop throughout life as our circumstances change.

As your child goes through this process, he gradually comes to construct his own self concepts by accumulating knowledge about his gender, appearance, race and physical, intellectual and interpersonal skills.

The First Five Years

Little by little, your child will move from a sense of his physical self to his social and emotional self to some understanding of his intellectual self. He will come to:

* Recognise images of himself.

* Establish whether he is a boy or a girl.

* Understand what age and race he is.

* Understand what he likes and does not like.

* Understand how well he can express and control his feelings.

* Establish how confident he feels about his ability at certain subjects, such as maths and English.

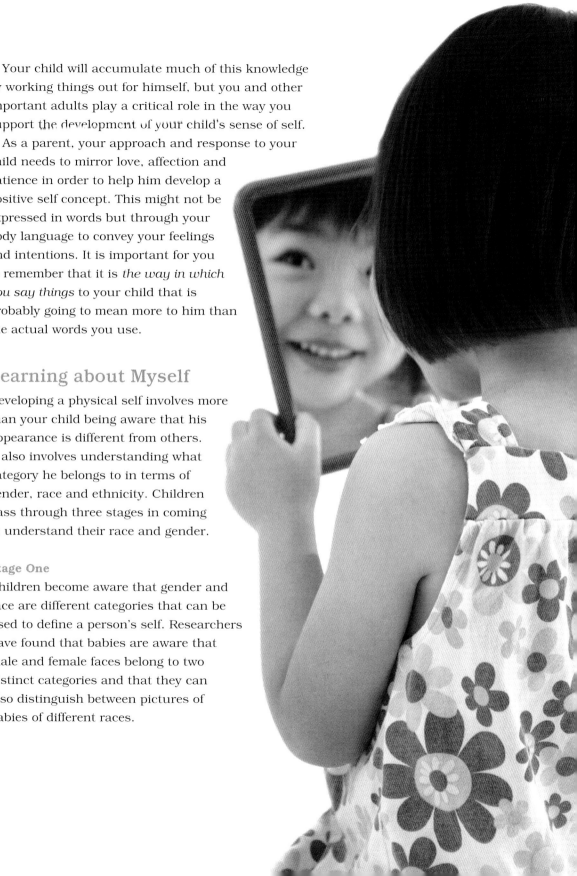

Your child will accumulate much of this knowledge by working things out for himself, but you and other important adults play a critical role in the way you support the development of your child's sense of self.

As a parent, your approach and response to your child needs to mirror love, affection and patience in order to help him develop a positive self concept. This might not be expressed in words but through your body language to convey your feelings and intentions. It is important for you to remember that it is *the way in which you say things* to your child that is probably going to mean more to him than the actual words you use.

Learning about Myself

Developing a physical self involves more than your child being aware that his appearance is different from others. It also involves understanding what category he belongs to in terms of gender, race and ethnicity. Children pass through three stages in coming to understand their race and gender.

Stage One

Children become aware that gender and race are different categories that can be used to define a person's self. Researchers have found that babies are aware that male and female faces belong to two distinct categories and that they can also distinguish between pictures of babies of different races.

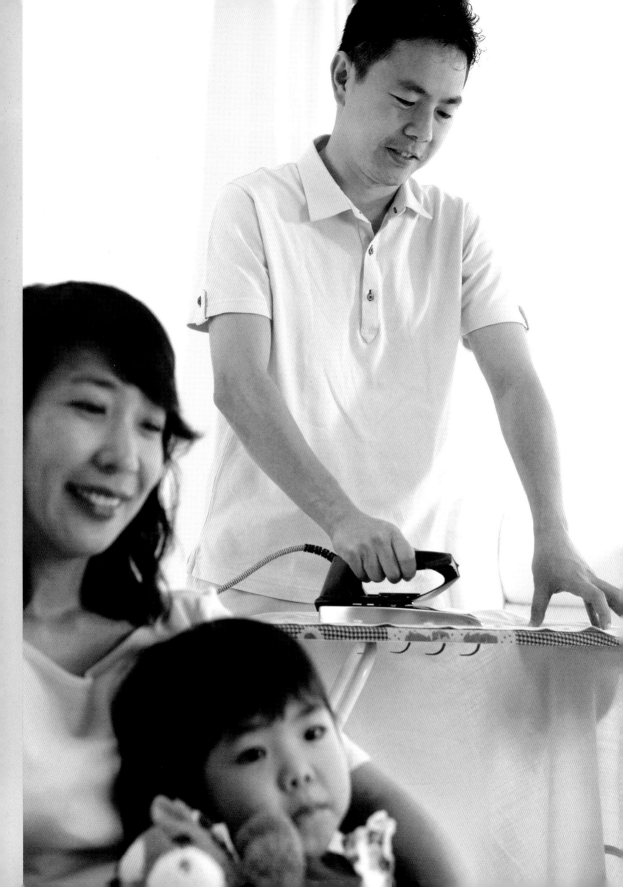

Stage Two

Between the ages of 2 and 3, children are able to identify and label their own sex and if asked whether they were a boy or girl when they were born, they are more likely to answer they were just a baby then, but now they are a boy/girl!

Stage Three

By the age of 5, children understand gender remains stable and that if you dress a boy doll in a pink dress, he will still be a boy. But research has found that children's understanding that race is constant and cannot change develops later than gender constancy.

Helping Your Child to Understand His Physical Self

* Dr Seuss' *My Book about Me* is a lovely book to use with toddlers to help them define their self concept. Paste your child's picture on the cover and discuss his appearance, gender, etc. There are other activities in the book, like tracing around feet and hands to see how big they are, which will appeal to children at this age and help to further establish their self concept.

* Make up your own book using small photo albums and insert photos of your child doing things with family and friends. Use these photos to talk about the differences and similarities between your child and others and how special he is. Continue to create these "Me" books on a regular basis. An alternative to "Me" books are home videos of your child and his friends.

Forming Gender Roles

A young child's view of what is typically masculine or feminine is limited to his experiences and he may form stereotypes of gender roles if that is the only exposure he has to this.

Give your child from the age of about 2½ the opportunity to role play at home to help him explore the different roles men and women play in society today.

A child's rigid stereotyping of how boys and girls should behave will become more relaxed if he sees both parents taking responsibility for care-giving and household duties.

Developing Self-control

The critical task facing your young child when developing his social and emotional self is to learn how to control his emotions. He needs to learn how to do things expected of him, even if he does not want to, and to cope with frustration and wait for what he wants. The child who cannot regulate his negative emotions, like anger and distress, runs the risk of being less successful at school.

Expressing and Controlling Feelings

Young children can experience very strong feelings that they find hard to express and control. Many parents have been faced with such embarrassing scenes when their children's behaviour challenges them in public.

Regulating the social self is not an easy task for young children. They have to learn how to adjust their feelings so they can successfully achieve their goals without over-stepping the boundaries of acceptable behaviour. Furthermore, they need to learn how to control both positive and negative feelings.

The Child's Temperament

Temperament plays an important role in accounting for the ways children differ in their emotional reactions, attention span, persistence and the ability to control their emotions. Children are born with different temperaments and this influences the way parents interact with them.

* Children born with more easy-going temperaments will find it easier to overcome emotional difficulties and will evoke more positive reactions from their parents.

* Children born with more difficult or slow-to-warm-up temperaments will be more vulnerable when trying to overcome emotional problems and will need sensitive parents who know when to push and when to back down in the face of their children's emotional outbursts.

The causes of children's tantrums change with the age and the stage they are at in terms of their emotional development. For example, what provoked a tantrum in an 18-month-old may not trigger such an outburst in a 3-year-old. Children are born unique and so there is no one prescription for parents to use when faced with a child having a full-blown tantrum.

How to Help Your Child Avoid or Recover from a Tantrum

* When your child experiences anger or fear, allow him to calm down, then talk about the situation with him. Ask him questions like "Why were you angry at dinner?", "Why do you think other people get angry?", "Do you understand why your sister got angry with you?" If you talk through these emotional experiences, your child is more likely to understand his feelings and the feelings of others. These talks provide a platform for you to help your child understand that there are alternatives to throwing a tantrum.

* Teach your child strategies to control his temper by introducing him to specific words or phrases he can use to express his anger instead of hitting out. For example, teach him key phrases like "I'm angry because you won't let me watch TV/play outside." By expanding his vocabulary to express his feelings, he can then describe what he feels, why he acted in a certain way and begin to gain mastery over his emotions.

* Constantly remind your child of new strategies and give him opportunities to practise them in everyday life situations.

* When your child shows acceptable behaviour, be sure to encourage and praise him.

* Reassure your child that he is still loved even if he shows negative ways of expressing his emotions. *Always focus on the unacceptable behaviour, never on the child!*

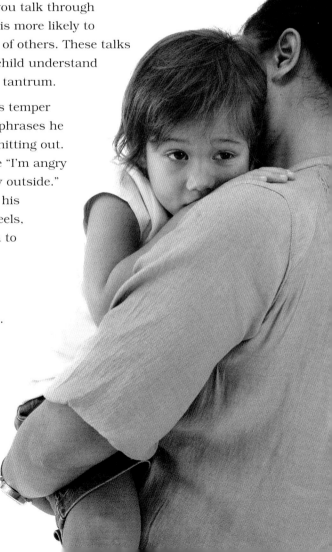

Developing Self-esteem

Your child needs to believe in himself, have confidence in his abilities and feel he is valued and loved by those around him. He needs, in other words, to develop self-esteem. This 'intellectual' self develops as your child interacts and forms relationships with you and other important people in his life. It is important for your child to develop high self-esteem in order to fulfil his potential. If he has positive feelings about himself, it will help him to take on new challenges, ask for help when he needs it and make friends more easily.

Praising Effort and Achievement

Remember to praise effort as well as achievement in order to avoid making your child feel that he is loved only when he succeeds.

Building Your Child's Confidence

You can play a critical role in helping your child develop high self-esteem by:

* Encouraging him to try new things and not to worry if he makes mistakes.

* Praising his effort and perseverance.

* Setting realistic expectations for him.

Do Not Over-praise or Criticise

Be cautious about over-praising your child for every task he succeeds in, even those that do not challenge him and telling him all the time that he is intelligent or clever to boost his self-esteem. This might make him overconfident and vulnerable to disappointment later on.

On the other hand, avoid criticising your child for what he cannot do. Help your child feel proud of who he is and what he has achieved. You are the key player in supporting and nurturing this process of your child's development from the physical to the social or emotional and the intellectual self.

Focus on Effort

Enthuse about the strategies your child is using and the perseverance and concentration he is showing, rather than focussing all the time on what he is actually achieving, because these are the vital skills he needs to become a more independent, competent and confident learner.

Allow Your Child to Make His Own Decisions

Don't always make decisions for your child. Young as he is, allow him to make certain choices like what to wear and what he wants to play with. All these will go a long way to help build your child's confidence and self-esteem.

Provide Consistent Love and Care

Provide consistent care for your child to help him feel secure, loved and valued for who he is, not what he does or how he looks like. This will also help him feel that he is special and worth other people spending time on him.

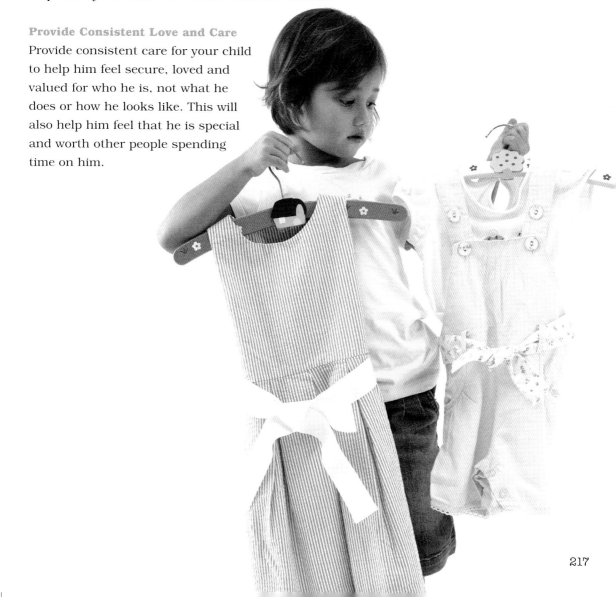

ENCOURAGE POSITIVE SELF-ESTEEM

☐ Say positive things to your child on a regular basis so he knows that you believe in him. Avoid using negative comparisons, for example, "Mark's so much slower than his brother in reading."

☐ Set realistic expectations and plan appropriate activities that are deserving of your child's time, ensuring that the tasks challenge and do not insult his abilities.

☐ Give meaningful feedback and help your child acknowledge what he can do without bragging.

☐ Express genuine interest in him and what he is doing.

☐ Encourage him to develop new skills which are not confined to formal learning. This can include household chores, such as setting the table or washing the car.

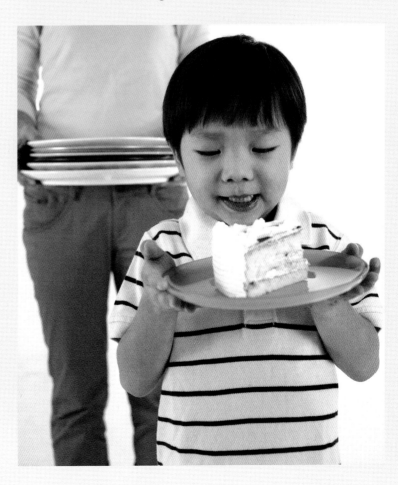

- [ ] Use encouragement and avoid empty praise.
- [ ] Allow him to make some decisions and choices to help develop greater independence.
- [ ] Give minimum assistance wherever possible in order to allow your child to maintain control over his activities.

TEACHING NEW SKILLS

New skills need to be taught. Children do not just catch on from watching. Don't expect your child to clear the table, make his bed or tidy up the room unless you have modelled the skills for him. Follow these steps to help your child to become independent.

Watch me	: You do most of the task, for example putting on shoes.
You help me	: You do less and encourage your child to do more.
I'll help you	: Your child does more but you stay to help and encourage.
I'll watch you	: Leave your child alone but check. Give encouragement on the progress he is making.

Adapted from *Positive Parenting* by Focus on the Family

Don't try to teach your child when you are under pressure or tired. You will end up nagging and scolding. You may need to work with other adults in the family to ensure they support you in this process.

Influence of Family

As parents, you have more influence over your child's development and identity than anyone else. From you, your child will learn about his family history and culture, and the kinds of social skills and behaviour that are appropriate and expected in his culture and environment.

Best Environment for Raising a Child

The family where there is a mother and a father present is recognised as the best environment for raising a child.

The family should be a secure environment where your child can learn to trust adults, where boundaries are set for his behaviour and where encouragement is given. The family should not only provide for your child's physical needs but also his social, emotional, intellectual, moral, spiritual and behavioural needs.

Special Role of Fathers

Although many fathers continue to work long hours, there is more awareness now among fathers of the importance of their role in the upbringing of their children. Studies show that children whose fathers play an active role in their lives are more likely to stay out of trouble and have a positive self-image.

Fathers are also important for developing a child's sex role identity. Children who have experienced both maleness and femaleness in their parents are more likely to be confident in this aspect of their development.

In all cultures, fathers are more likely to indulge in rough play with their children, which results in children being better able to react to stress and change. Boys in particular learn how to get excited and yet not hurt themselves and others, as fathers monitor the safety of the play and impose some rules. Fathers tend to do more outdoor activities with children, urging them to try harder and be more daring. As a result of this physical exercise, children sleep better and become better coordinated. Rising to physical challenges— provided these are realistic—gives a boost to their self-esteem.

Domestic Helpers

In Asia, the availability of domestic help for child care eases the pressures on parents. Sometimes, working parents can be jealous that their child is fond of the carer or filled with anxiety if the child seems unhappy. It is important to recognise these feelings and address them because, for the sake of the child, it is better that everyone likes and trusts one another.

Grandparents

Grandchildren are often eagerly anticipated and grandparents are sometimes prepared to stop working to care for their grandchildren. Unlike domestic helpers, they are not likely to leave the job unless they fall ill and so provide more stability —something that is especially important in the child's early years.

Arrangements where grandparents look after the child during the day in the working week, and parents take over at night seem to work well.

Unlike domestic helpers, grandparents share the same family background and family history and usually the same family languages. By virtue of this, they can ensure that children maintain the family, cultural and religious practices that form part of their identity.

Setting the Rules

Should your parents, parents-in-law or a child minder be the main caregiver for your child, ensure that you have an agreement about routines and behaviour management or your child will find it easy to play one side against the other. Be prepared, however, to give your child's grandparents some licence for treats by virtue of the fact that they are the grandparents.

PARENTING STYLES

You and your spouse may have experienced different parenting styles and have different ideas about what is appropriate. For the sake of your child and your marriage relationship, it is a good idea that you come to some agreement about how to bring up your child before he arrives. If it is too late for that, at the very least, it is important that you support each other in decisions made in front of your child.

The three main styles of parenting are detailed below.

Authoritarian Parenting

Parents who are authoritarians have high expectations of their child, exert control and set firm limits that are non-negotiable and may not be explained.

Permissive Parenting

Permissive parents do not take control. They allow the child plenty of freedom and choice.

Authoritative Parenting

Authoritative parents fall somewhere between authoritarian parents and permissive parents. Authoritative parents set rules or boundaries which help their child to feel secure and know that his parents care. They also consistently enforce these rules while giving their child the reasons for doing so. They give choices, listen to their child and, as the child gets older, allow for negotiation.

WHICH STYLE IS BEST?

The authoritative parenting style is generally thought to be the best for children as it produces the following outcomes: children are well adjusted, friendly with peers and co-operative with adults. They have high self-esteem, develop independence and display good self-control.

In Asia, emphasis is placed on authoritarian parenting and children do well because of the consistent approach and high expectations of behaviour. This authoritarian style of parenting should strike a balance between 'soft' love and 'firm' love; love being the motivating factor for being warm with your child so he feels cared for and supported, and also for being firm, so he knows who is in control and will learn to respect and trust you.

Don't set too high a standard for yourself as a parent. Parenting is a role in which you can feel like a failure at times, but children thrive with a 'good enough' parenting style where there is consistency in their care and love is shown to them. Family therapists suggest trusting your instincts as a parent, doing what is right for you and getting practical help when you need it.

A SUPPORTIVE HOME ENVIRONMENT

Your home has a major impact on your child's development and socialisation. Ideally, the home should be a place where your child can:

☐ Practise social skills and develop confidence.

☐ Play with and learn from others.

☐ Develop a sense of responsibility so that he feels useful.

☐ Converse with others so his interests and opinions can be respectfully shared and his questions answered.

☐ Have some privacy and space for play. Storage for his possessions should take into account his age and stage of development, without excessive and inappropriate demands for tidiness. (That said, your child's needs should not override the needs of adults in the family for space and relaxation.)

☐ Learn to understand his culture and important practices.

☐ Be given appropriate praise and encouragement to motivate him to improve his skills and knowledge.

☐ Manage his behaviour and grow in independence and self discipline with limits that are set to help him achieve this.

With subsequent children, you may be more relaxed or more stretched. Whatever it is, if you want the best for your children, keep yourself motivated as you parent more children.

Communicate with your children and be aware about how they feel about themselves and each other.

Having this kind of 'health check' will allow you to make adjustments in the way you treat your children, leading to happier and healthier relationships within the family.

THE CHILD'S POSITION IN THE FAMILY

Does a child's position in the family affect their personality traits? For example, does a middle child often fit the label of "difficult", the oldest the label of "hardworking" and "responsible" and the youngest the label of "most extrovert", "creative" or "naughty"?

The Firstborn

It is easy to see that firstborns have the initial advantage of being the only child for some time, having more personal attention, and more of the available resources parents can afford or offer. As the family increases in size, they are less likely to be overindulged, a criticism often levelled at the only child. As the eldest, they may well be given more responsibility and parents' expectations of them may be higher. Part of this responsibility may be to tutor younger brothers and sisters, and this improves verbal and cognitive skills. This learning-by-teaching pays dividends in later life, making them leaders rather than followers.

The Only Child

Increasingly, being an only child is the experience of many. The only child may initially be less socially skilled in playing with other children as he has fewer opportunities for sharing and playing with others, but appears to be just as socially competent later on. He may, however, be more mature in his communication skills—the 'little old man'—as he relates more to adults in the family than children. He is likely to have higher self-esteem, enjoy a closer relationship with his parents and do better academically.

Being the sole focus of parents, and maybe even grandparents, can, but need not, place undue pressure on the child to succeed. It is a more lonely life, without the highs and lows of conflict and caring that siblings bring, and later with no one to share the care of elderly parents. Initially, however, the child benefits materially and in terms of privacy, time and attention.

Twins

Twins are often slower to speak as they develop their own private means of communication and by virtue of their being a pair, they get less individual attention from adults. They may often be referred to as "the twins" and if they look alike and parents choose to dress them alike, it is important to remember that their own individual and unique identities still need to be recognised.

The Middle Child

The middle child lacks the status of being the eldest and may be denied the special treatment the youngest child gets. This can be the reason why the middle child is sometimes labelled as difficult. However, much will depend on how the child reacts to this. Middle children are also described as helpful, sociable and affectionate!

The Youngest Child

There are a diverse set of descriptors that have been used for youngest children ranging from attention-seeking, sensitive, affectionate, indulged, charming, sociable, relaxed and rebellious. Much depends on the parents, the personality of the child, the size of the family and the gap between the last child and the previous one. Sometimes the last child can be the long awaited boy or girl or conversely a 'mistake' and this influences the way the child is treated.

Some parents see the youngest child as their last chance to do things right. They pin all their hopes on this child. In this case, the child can be under a great deal of pressure to perform and behave. More often, however, the youngest child is under less pressure—in large families, and where parents are older, they may adopt a less intense and more relaxed attitude.

By virtue of being the youngest, the child may receive more help and protection from parents and may take advantage of his position to become manipulative. He, and not his older brother or sister, may be the provoker in sibling relationships. Depending on his relationships with his siblings and how they perceive their parents treat them, he may be protected and helped or resented by them. Those who have been the youngest child talk about feeling a lack of status—always having hand-me-downs instead of new things. If frequently compared to older siblings, they speak of finding it hard to measure up. Depending on personality and the treatment the child receives, he may resent being treated as the 'baby' in the family or enjoy it as a favoured position.

Family Models

The behaviour your child sees modelled within the family has a powerful influence on him. It will help him form perceptions of gender roles and impact how he sees himself and relates to others.

Shared Roles

If the roles within your household are shared or less distinct (you and your spouse share household tasks and child care, and contribute to the family finances), your child will benefit from the variety of carers and may have a closer relationship with his father. In the long term, he may also be more open to taking on roles and jobs that suit his personality and skills rather than his gender.

Shared roles also allow the mother more time to enjoy her children and follow some of her own interests. The quality of the marriage is also said to improve.

Traditional Roles

If the roles within your household are traditional (the father makes the big, financial decisions and seldom participates in housework or child care, and the mother performs more household tasks and plays a greater part in child care), your son may have a tougher time when he has to fend for himself, for example when studying overseas or entering the army.

Where roles are reversed and the father takes on the responsibility of the carer while the mother becomes the financial provider, research has shown that there is no effect on the children, provided that the father—and mother—are confident of the father's worth and skills in managing the children.

Sexual Roles

The sexual roles your child adopts are influenced by physical factors like hormones, but also by the way he is brought up, such as the toys he is given, the way he is dressed, by what he observes of men and women within the family and society, what he sees in books, newspapers, magazines and on TV and whether distinct male and female roles are encouraged or discouraged by the adults around him.

Fathers

Fathers play an important role in the development of their children's sex role identity. It has been found that fathers can be more rigid than mothers about enforcing specific gender roles, especially with boys—like scolding them for crying, expecting them to be braver than girls and being less open than mothers in allowing their sons to play with dolls. This is a contentious area and you have every right to decide how to bring up your children. But fathers should be aware of their role in moulding the feelings and compassionate side of their sons' characters.

Other Influences

Domestic Helpers

Other role models within the home that exert an influence on children are the domestic helpers, whether full- or part-time. Select your domestic helper with care and take the time to train and orientate her to your ways, values and expectations for your child.

Children are manipulative. If left unchecked, they can take advantage of your helper's position and fail to develop the necessary independence and responsibility.

Not only will your child learn from your helper, he will also learn from the way you treat her. Treating your helper as a person and ensuring your exchanges with her are pleasant and respectful will go a long way towards educating your child about how he should relate to and treat others.

Neighbours

Neighbours and others in the community can also become supportive helpers to your family in times of need. Treat your neighbours as you would have them treat you. It is good for your child to see this behaviour modelled and absorb it as a principle and as a part of his moral code for relationships within the family and with others in the community.

Preschoolers and Gender Roles

Preschoolers go through a period of being rigid about what is appropriate and what is not appropriate for males and females. They are less rigid after the age of 7.

Parents and preschool teachers can help by providing books, activities and schedules that give boys and girls equal opportunities and encouragement to participate in, for example, building bricks, block play and home play, and placing less emphasis on models that are sex stereotypes.

Girls need opportunities to develop their spatial skills as much as boys need opportunities to develop the caring side of their personalities.

In difficult situations such as the loss of a parent or when there is parental conflict, divorce or remarriage, children can be a source of great emotional support for one another. In spite of their protests, children often enjoy the thrill of riling and annoying a sibling! However, there are other benefits too.

- The older child provides support for his younger siblings.
- The older child benefits from the chance to develop responsibility, teach, share and protect his younger siblings.
- The younger child has a companion, a helper and someone to learn from.
- There is a positive impact on the child's moral maturity and relationships with other children.

SIBLING RELATIONSHIPS

Sibling relationships can be close or marked by conflict. Whichever way, they provide frequent opportunities for interaction and learning. Through these relationships, your children learn how to comfort, share and co-operate as well as to deceive, manipulate, annoy and argue.

Unless the gap between siblings is a big one, some squabbling or conflict is inevitable. This is stressful to you and your spouse, and you can be drawn in to giving attention to the squabbling by shouting, threatening or taking sides. While it is tempting to blame the older child, be aware that younger children can be the cause of the problem.

An age gap of two to four years appears to lead to more conflict and rivalry because siblings born this close together are so similar in needs and development. However, the most important factor in determining how children get along together seems to be their individual temperaments or personalities and how these fit together. Similarly, with regard to sibling relationships, personality is more important than birth order.

Sorting Out Conflicts

Unless your children are in danger of inflicting serious injury on one another, leave them to sort out their own squabbles, giving them due notice that this is what you are going to do. As trying as these situations are, it is consoling to know that children are learning about what causes conflict, how it works and, hopefully, how to manage it and negotiate solutions.

Same-sex Siblings

Have you ever wondered whether there is more conflict between children of the same or different sex? Research has found that generally, there is more conflict and more aggression between same-sex siblings but same-sex siblings can also be extremely close to one another.

LOSING AN ATTACHMENT FIGURE

Losing an attachment figure like a grandparent or a domestic helper can be traumatic for a child. Where parents work, the child may spend long hours with a grandparent or helper and develop attachments to these people that may be stronger than attachments to his parents.

When a helper leaves, the attachment bond is broken and the child can become distraught. Sometimes, parents can be at a loss as to how to manage and comfort the child. Since consistency is important in building attachments and trust, it is important for parents to spend time developing their own attachments with the child and to try to avoid changing helpers too frequently.

Children have very limited experience of loss and death and sometimes a parent's own grief can mean that the child's grief is left unaddressed. This can lead to behavioural problems as the child acts up as a cry for help. Again the situation needs to be addressed in terms of what the child can understand, and since grief is a process rather than a one-time event, it will need to be addressed and readdressed.

Family Time

Planning regular family times is a good idea for developing togetherness and imparting your values to your child. These sessions can be as simple as watching a TV programme, playing a board game or going for a walk together.

Mealtime Lessons

Take the opportunity at mealtimes to model and teach your child good table manners and impart healthy eating habits.

Mealtimes can also be made more fun by letting your child decide on the menu and help in the preparation. He can also help with decorating the table for special occasions like birthdays.

Eating Together

If both you and your spouse work on different schedules and return home late, you probably have little time to have a meal together as a family. While this may be the case during the working week, try having a meal together at least once a week at the weekend. For this meal, every family member should be seated at the table with the TV turned off so that there are opportunities for conversation.

Family Discussions

Family discussions can take place over dinner and topics can include things you are about to purchase for your child, like a bicycle or a computer, where to go and what to do on the upcoming public holiday, or bigger issues like where to spend the next family holiday.

Introducing Simple Rules

It helps to introduce some simple rules like listening to everyone's ideas, starting with the oldest person and taking turns. Discussing or talking about issues like what you can afford and whether it is sensible to spend time and money on a particular item teach your child the value of money.

Parents or elders have the final say but giving your child the opportunity to discuss such matters shows your child that his opinions are valued. He may also begin to see that interesting and fun things to do need not be expensive.

Relaxing Together

Factoring in times in the day once or twice a week to relax with your child is important and goes a long way to show him that he is valued.

* Go for a walk.

* Watch TV.

* Play a card or board game.

* Give your child a bath.

* Do the bedtime routine with **story time built in**.

* Chat about the events of the day.

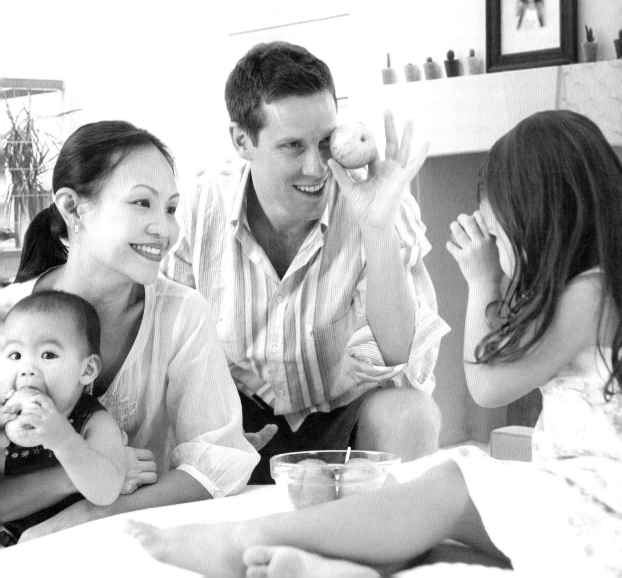

Family Rituals

Family rituals consisting of birthdays and special celebrations, traditions and routines give your child a sense of belonging and security. Young children thrive on repetition and yet love surprises too. Some of these are times when you can naturally build in your personal values and impart them to your child.

Birthdays

Celebrating your child's birthday provides the opportunity to enjoy some family time together while helping him to feel loved and showing him that you value his growing maturity.

Celebrating birthdays also provides a significant marker for change. For example, you can use this opportunity to clear out the toys and clothing that your child has outgrown and re-arrange his room. You can also use this milestone to expect changes in behaviour like a dry bed at night and settling his own squabbles with siblings or friends, and to start having pocket money.

Involve your child in planning the actual celebration whether it is for himself or for others in the family.

Special Celebrations

Let your child choose and put up decorations, and help to prepare some of the special food.

Talk to him about the special food and practices that mark these celebrations, like giving gifts and putting on new clothes, and their significance. Teach him acceptable behaviour such as greeting others, saying "Thank you" for presents and not opening gifts in front of the giver.

Your Everyday Lifestyle

In the same way that children remember feelings more than words, your child is more likely to follow what he sees you do—how you spend your time and money, and how you treat others—than what you say. He will learn to respect and value people and to be forgiving if he sees it modelled.

* Show compassion and care for others when they are ill, hurt or upset, in your family, in your child's class or in the community by visiting or calling. Get your child to draw a picture or make a card for the person.

* Treat others with respect such as saying "Please", "Thank you" and "I'm sorry". This includes your spouse, your parents and in-laws, your domestic helper, people of other cultures and faiths, people with disabilities and your own children.

* Have a sense of wonder and thankfulness. Encourage this by pointing out things in the natural world to your child. Allow your child to touch them and help him to appreciate how they look, sound, smell and feel. If you have a particular fear or dislike for insects, cockroaches, geckos etc., try not to pass it on to your child.

* Answer your child's questions. "Why did the bird die?", "How does a baby get inside his mummy's tummy?" Answer at his level and when you do not know, be truthful and say that you do not know. Read a book together to discover the answer.

* Lead by example, such as by observing a healthy lifestyle by paying attention to your health, eating sensibly and exercising.

* Attitudes to life can be infectious so model being contented, happy and optimistic. Some children are particularly prone to griping about what they have to do and what they cannot have. These children need to know that happiness is a choice and need not be dependent on circumstances.

* Show your child how to appreciate peace and quietness by insisting on a quiet home some of the time. It is important for your child to know how to appreciate quietness and be able to entertain himself by playing or reading quietly. By doing so, he will develop concentration and perhaps a more reflective disposition.

* Let your child know that your love is not conditional on good behaviour and success. Point out that you do not always love what he does but you still love him. Encourage him to know what he can do about mistakes by learning from them, saying sorry and adopting a problem-solving attitude to doing something about changing.

Moral Development

Your child is not born with a moral conscience. You and the other members of your family need to be the moral compass guiding him in developing his moral values and behaviour. Your child will look to you, in particular, to clearly define and model moral values, and to set the boundaries for him so he can understand right from wrong.

Knowing Right from Wrong

Your child will be able to distinguish between different types of rules by the age of 5. For example, he will understand that it is wrong to hit someone because you may hurt them. Even young children who are not yet able to talk are capable of learning a great deal about cause and effect by experiencing first-hand what makes people angry and what their reactions will be. For example, taking away a toy another child is playing with or throwing his bowl on the floor when he is not allowed to eat any more ice cream is not acceptable.

In such situations, guide your child through discussions to negotiate with others (rather than manipulate) in order to reach an amicable agreement. It will help your child see what went wrong and how it could be handled better the next time.

Identifying and Dealing with Emotions

One important aspect of moral development and general well-being is the ability to identify both positive and negative emotions like anger, jealousy, disgust, pride, humiliation, disappointment and shame, and knowing how to deal with them.

* Seize teachable moments to discuss positive and negative feelings with your child and the desirable behaviour he can use to express or contain these emotions.

* Consistently act according to the values you profess to hold. Your child needs to see you practise what you preach. If your child is brought up by multiple caregivers whose behaviour does not reflect their so-called values, your child will become confused. It is therefore crucial for you to make sure everyone is on the same page when it comes to doing what they say they believe in.

Telling Lies

Some parents are troubled when their children tell lies. They feel that they have failed to inculcate the correct moral values in their children. Nothing could be further from the truth. Research has shown that children under 4 years old do not understand that other people have minds and can think thoughts like they do. They also cannot understand that other people will see things from a different point of view to theirs.

Helen, 3 years old

Helen's mother hears a loud crash in the kitchen and rushes in to find her daughter surrounded by fragments of a dish that had obviously been broken while she was trying to reach for sweets on the shelf. When Helen sees her mother, she whispers, "The wind blew it off the shelf!"

Before deciding whether Helen was consciously trying to conceal the truth about the broken dish and whether she should be punished for lying, consider what lying involves.

A lie is an attempt to manipulate what you believe others are thinking to alter their belief to something false in order to protect yourself. But Helen is too young to understand what her mother is thinking. She is probably describing the situation as she wishes it had occurred, and that is not the same as concealing the truth. Rather than punishing Helen for her "lie", it would be better for her parents to talk to her about the consequences involved in touching things without asking permission.

With an older child who can figure out what others are thinking and is aware he is telling lies, the discussion would need to involve words like "meant to", "accidentally", "on purpose" and "mistake" to establish how culpable the child was for the deed. And, if indeed, the child is lying, avoid saying things like:

* You are bad.

* You are naughty.

* I don't love you anymore.

Instead, convey the following messages:

* I did not like what you did.

* I appreciate you tried to clear up.

* I still love you in spite of the mistake you made.

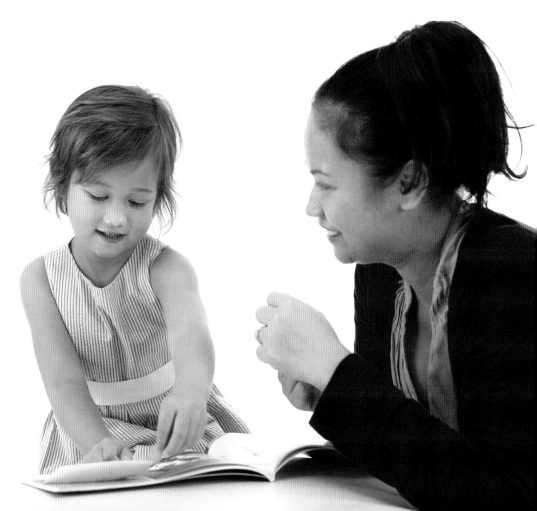

Be aware and careful not to scold your child constantly for everything that he does wrong. Your child will start to feel bad about himself and run the risk of having low self-esteem. He is also less likely to be highly developed morally as he will be unable to move beyond his own needs to respecting and valuing those of others.

Aggression

Psychologists suggest that the child who behaves in an aggressive, anti-social manner may also be limited in his ability to view things from another person's perspective and thus lag behind in his moral understanding.

He may also have high self-esteem and over-estimate his competence. If the adults in his life have not taken steps to explain and demonstrate that aggression is morally unacceptable, he will continue to use such behaviour to get his way.

This is especially so if the child has witnessed aggression at home and seen that it works. But aggression may not always be dealt with at home as many children only exhibit such behaviour when they are in competition with other children at school.

Family members need to devalue aggressive behaviour and take the lead to help the child find morally acceptable ways of getting what he wants and realising his goals.

Ability to Judge Intentions

In order to develop a moral conscience and understand the difference between right and wrong, your child needs to be able to judge whether someone intended to do something wrong and see the consequences of that action.

As the example with Helen discussed above shows, younger children are not capable of projecting into other people's minds to assess whether their intentions are morally correct or not. It is therefore important that you do not automatically accuse your child of doing something wrong and punish him. Make allowances for the natural limitations of your child's thinking abilities and respond appropriately to them.

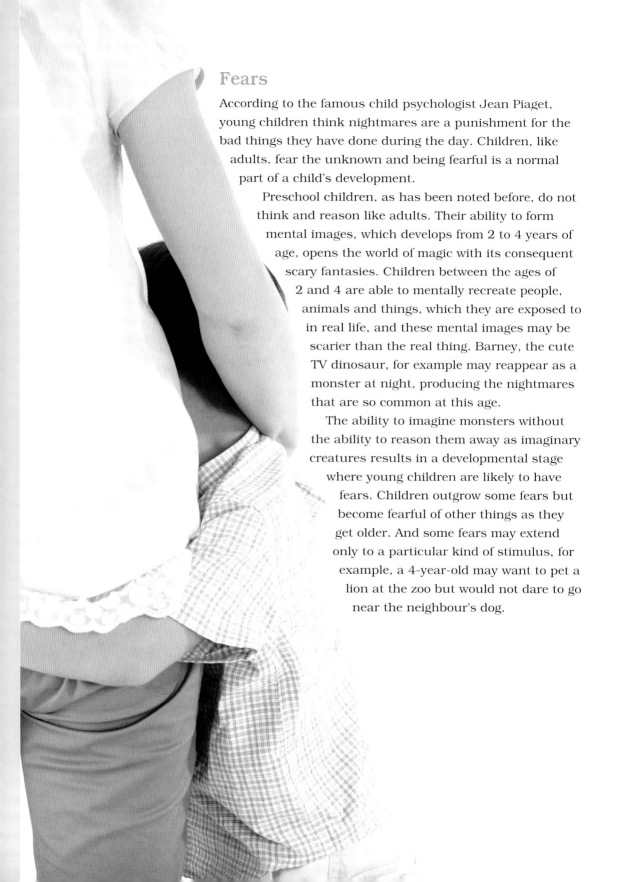

Fears

According to the famous child psychologist Jean Piaget, young children think nightmares are a punishment for the bad things they have done during the day. Children, like adults, fear the unknown and being fearful is a normal part of a child's development.

Preschool children, as has been noted before, do not think and reason like adults. Their ability to form mental images, which develops from 2 to 4 years of age, opens the world of magic with its consequent scary fantasies. Children between the ages of 2 and 4 are able to mentally recreate people, animals and things, which they are exposed to in real life, and these mental images may be scarier than the real thing. Barney, the cute TV dinosaur, for example may reappear as a monster at night, producing the nightmares that are so common at this age.

The ability to imagine monsters without the ability to reason them away as imaginary creatures results in a developmental stage where young children are likely to have fears. Children outgrow some fears but become fearful of other things as they get older. And some fears may extend only to a particular kind of stimulus, for example, a 4-year-old may want to pet a lion at the zoo but would not dare to go near the neighbour's dog.

Fears at Different Ages

Age	Fears
3 years	Loud noises, the dark, thunder and lightning, toilet training, animals, doctors, strangers and separation, animals who look odd (larger-than-life puppets at the Chingay Parade for example)
4 to 5 years	All of the above, plus fears about things that are not real, like monsters and ghosts for example and animals, like dogs.
6 to 7 years	Children's fears are more concrete about things that could happen to them. For example, divorce of parents, health issues, being injured (being hit by a car for example) and natural disasters.

Irrational Fears

Does your child have phobias that seem irrational for his age and developmental level, and do these fears interfere with his daily activities?

For example, while it is quite normal for a 2-year-old to be afraid of sitting on a potty, it is not so for a 6-year-old.

Seek assistance from a child psychologist if you find that your child is developing such phobias.

Night-time Fears

Fear of the Dark and Separation Anxiety

Fear of the dark and of separation from parents is a double fear that keeps many children awake. Most children are afraid of the dark and if they have encountered fantasy characters, like monsters and ghosts in stories or on TV/films, this will heighten their fear, even if they have night lights in their rooms.

A child's ability to distinguish appearances from reality, together with the understanding that he will see his loved ones again in the morning, and his ability to better control his feelings of panic or anxiety only develop around the ages of 5 or 6.

Leaving Children to Cry It Out

Many parents, in line with more Western beliefs, are often advised to let their child cry out his fears alone in his bedroom at night.

Young children do not have the coping strategies to deal with the panic they feel at being left alone and such an approach for young babies and children who are particularly fearful or anxious is not appropriate.

Sleeping Together and Co-sleeping

Parents who do not believe in letting their child sleep alone at night sometimes arrange for their child to sleep in their bedroom or co-sleep with siblings or a live-in domestic helper. Such arrangements go some way towards solving the problem of night-time fears.

For the child who sleeps alone in his own bedroom, however, parents can follow a bedtime ritual of lying down with him until he falls asleep. This can carry on until the child is old enough to enjoy going to sleep on his own.

An alternative solution is to leave the light on in the bedroom until the child is comfortable sleeping in the dark.

Suggestions for Helping Your Child Cope with Night-time Fears

Whatever sleeping arrangements are made, your child needs to be assured that he is safe and secure when the lights go out and that someone will be there to respond sympathetically to his night-time fears. This will not only ease your child's anxieties, it will also provide an opportunity to strengthen your relationship with him. As you work together with your child through his fears, he will learn to regard you as a valuable source of support.

* Be aware that daytime stressors can play on your child's mind at night. For example, having no friends at preschool or being bullied. Discuss these issues with your child during the day to relieve his stress.

* Avoid sending your child to bed too early. If he lies awake in his room, he is likely to dwell on his fears. Monitor, over a period of time, how much sleep your child usually needs and review his bedtime if necessary.

* Be selective about what your child watches or reads before sleeping. A recent study revealed that children aged 5 to 6 who watched adult programmes including the news, or were even just in the room passively listening, had more disturbed sleep and slept less overall. Help your child go to sleep with comforting bedtime rituals like a soothing story, massage or song. Play soothing music for an hour or so after your child falls asleep.

* If your child has a nightmare, break the spell by reacting immediately. Hug and comfort him and help him to think happy thoughts, such as playing with his favourite pet, or have him practise telling himself that he is brave.

* Don't ridicule your child's fears and say things like "Stop being a baby" or ignore the things he is afraid of. This may only drive your child's fears underground.

* Never use other fears to discipline your child by saying things like "The boogie man will come and get you!"

* Talk about his fears especially if there has been an event beforehand that has triggered the fears, and empathise with him. Confess, for example, that you were scared of dogs when you were his age but be careful not to get over-involved in your child's fears or be overprotective, as he may play on them to get your attention.

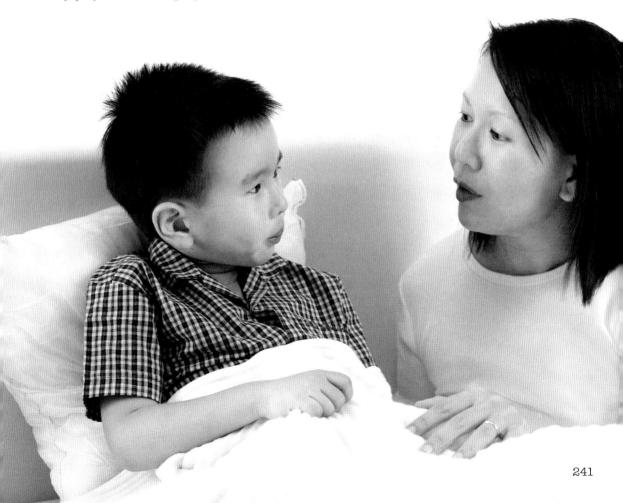

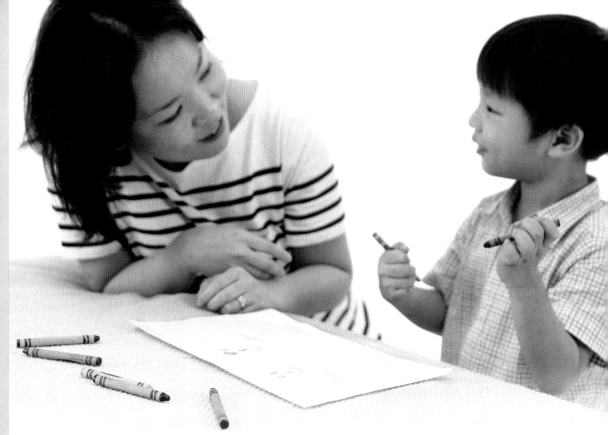

* Try to help him master his fears and reassure him that he will be okay. For example, if he is scared about going to school, say "I know you are scared of starting a new school and not having any friends, but you will feel much better once you get there and start to get to know other children, just like you've done before in new places." It may also be helpful to model or role play how he can go up and introduce himself to new people. Role playing can also be used to overcome night-time fears as well. You can play the role of the supportive parent while your child plays the scared child and then coming up with the different strategies to help him cope.

* Do not show your fears. Many children inherit their parents' fears if they see them over-reacting, such as the fear that many adults have of cockroaches.

* If your child is 4 years or older, work out his fears by drawing. For example, if your child fears the dark, ask him what his dark room feels like and looks like. If you get a black sheet of paper with an orange monster under the bed, you have pinpointed the fear.

TRY CREATING STORIES

Tell a story to your child during the day which can desensitise him of his fears by making him confront them in small steps.

Choose your child's favourite hero as the main character who has to learn to overcome his fear of cockroaches, for example.

Bob is busy digging a hole in the ground for a new pond in Mrs Tan's garden. It is very hot and he is feeling very tired.

He sits down in his van to take a rest when suddenly he sees a small cockroach crawling out of the hole he's dug in the garden. He is terrified!

He takes a deep breath to try and calm himself and shuts his eyes tightly.

When he opens them again, the cockroach is gone!

Bob heaves a huge sigh of relief. He picks up his spade and returns to his digging.

Out of the corner of his eye, he sees another cockroach crawling around but he ignores it and it slowly disappears.

Bob finishes digging the hole and goes home to rest and watch his favourite TV programme.

Boundaries for Behaviour

Your child is not born with an understanding of the rules of behaviour or knowledge of what is safe and unsafe. He has to learn them with your help. To be accepted in society and make friends, your child needs to have good manners; know how to greet others, particularly elders; share and cooperate with others and say "Please" and "Thank you".

Children Learn What They Live with

Children watch to see how behaviour is received and begin to work out what is acceptable. They adapt their behaviour to the setting so you will find that your child can be very different in behaviour at home and at school. Limits need to be realistic for your child's age and also agreed within the family so your child knows where he stands.

Disciplining Your Child

Some children, by virtue of their temperament, will be easier or harder to manage and an approach that worked with one child may not work with another.

You may find that you have to cope with behaviour in a second or subsequent child that is very different from what you encountered with your first child. As each child is a unique individual, this is not really surprising, but it takes many parents by surprise.

Your Temperament Versus Your Child's

Be aware of your own temperament which may clash with your child's and lead to a battle of wills. There may also be particular times of the day when your child is more at risk of poor behaviour. These are usually around bedtime when your child is tired, before meals when he is hungry or when there is a change of routine or new people at home.

Instilling Self-discipline

The goal of discipline with children is self-discipline, meaning that your child will be able to behave and discipline himself when you are not around.

Young children, however, lack the ability to control themselves and only develop self-control or self-discipline by being controlled from the outside first. If boundaries or limits imposed on their behaviour are consistently applied, these give them a sense of security. They will test these boundaries and cannot be expected to behave well all of the time. Sometimes, a child's challenging and difficult behaviour can be because the boundaries are not realistic for the child's age or stage of development. At other times, challenging or difficult behaviour can be:

* To seek attention.

* The result of a power struggle between you and your child.

* To seek revenge.

* To show inadequacy. Your child is frustrated because he is facing a difficulty, such as dressing himself.

Parents sometimes react by shouting, scolding, nagging, making empty threats, coaxing, bribing or smacking. By giving the behaviour this kind of attention, these parents 'reward' it and so it tends to keep on happening.

Depending on your parenting style, the three approaches you can take to overcome such challenging or difficult behaviour are:

* The passive parenting approach—Give in.

* The aggressive parenting approach—Get harsh.

* The firm but kind parenting approach—Stay firm, positive and respectful. This takes more discipline on your part but is a positive approach that works best.

Positive Discipline

Set Reasonable Age-appropriate Limits or Boundaries and Stick to Them

Your child will test limits to see whether you remain firm but he does not expect you to give way. Remain firm but friendly, giving your reasons.

Your child will start being able to understand reasons when he is 3 to 4 years old and this corresponds with the time he begins to ask "Why".

Limits or boundaries should change as your child gets older and be negotiated in order to encourage independence and responsibility. In setting boundaries:

* Use clear, simple language.

* Remind your child about the boundaries you have set.

* Explain the limits so your child understands them.

* Praise your child when he behaves appropriately.

* Explain to your child what will happen when the limits are compromised. For example, if he continues to bang the table with the toy, the toy will be taken away.

Use "I" Messages

It is important to remember that the goal is to correct your child's behaviour and not to attack your child. So instead of using an accusing tone and saying things like "You're so clumsy/noisy" or "You little liar", let your child know how you feel by expressing your feelings in acceptable ways. You can do this by using "I" messages which will allow you to:

* Say what you feel—"I am upset that you spilt the juice."

* Say what you need—"I need you to get the cloth."

* Say what your position is—"I want you to clean it up."

"I" messages need to be delivered in as calm a manner as possible. The goal is to teach your child healthy ways of dealing with feelings like anger and solving problems, and how to cope with conflict since he will not always get his own way and cannot go throwing a toddler tantrum when he is grown up. Of course the most important "I" message is, "I'm sorry..."

Use Choices and Consequences

Giving your child the opportunity to make a choice can avoid you getting into a battle of wills, while making him feel that he has some control in a situation. Choices should be limited and whichever choice a child makes should be acceptable to you as the parent.

As your child gets older, he should be given choices in more areas, for example, in how to organise his time or spend his pocket money, but these come with corresponding responsibility.

If an "I" message does not work, you can try offering limited choices and letting your child live with the consequences of his choice—unless there is danger. Adults learn from the consequences of their behaviour such as overspending and procrastinating, and from young, your child too can learn from the consequences of his choices.

Here are some important points to note about using choices:

* Choices must be limited. For example, rice or noodles, a big spoonful or a small spoonful.

* Choices must be followed through. For example, "You wanted the noodles. You can have fruit as soon as you have eaten two more spoonfuls of noodles."

* Choices must be seen as a choice and not as a punishment. If your child cannot choose, you can say, "Then I will have to decide for you."

* Stay positive, calm and confident. Use phrases like "Yes, as soon as..." and "If you... you can..."

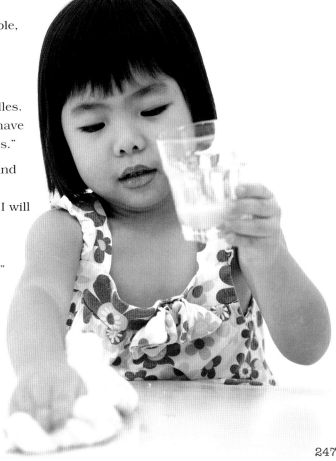

"I'm Sorry"

Is there any value in your child apologising if he does not mean it and does not sound as if he means it by his tone of voice? Experts feel that there is, as it is a public admission and acceptance of having done something wrong and brings the matter to some conclusion, although you should have your child do more to make amends.

* Consequences should flow naturally from the situation. If your child does not finish his food, he cannot have fruit or dessert. Consequences can be hard to think up! Give yourself time and ask your child to help you by asking, "What do you think we should do about this?"

* Leave room for a new start by saying something like "You can try again tomorrow."

The plus point about positive discipline is that it tells your child how he should be behaving as there is the expectation that he has to do something positive as a consequence of his negative behaviour.

The child who is rude is expected to apologise; the child who breaks things is expected to mend them or save up to replace them; the child who is mean or unkind to another person is expected to do something kind and helpful for that person; the child who is disobedient or irresponsible is given a task where he has to be responsible or especially obedient. You can add to this by telling your child why you have taken action by saying something like "I care about you so..."

Some Useful Tools

While it can be difficult for very young children to control their impulses to have or do something, they are easily distracted and so you can use distraction to get your child to refocus on something else. As children get older, they are less easy to distract and other methods are called for.

Ignoring and Giving Attention

Ignoring can be a sound technique for preschool and older children, provided that they are not at risk of hurting themselves or others. Any form of attention is rewarding for a child and the theory is that if the misbehaviour is ignored, it will diminish. In most cases this is so, but some children will continue until they find something that cannot be ignored and then they need to be given a choice to stop the behaviour or face the consequences.

When you give your child your attention, it shows him that he is valued. When he is working well at something and putting in effort, take an interest in what he is doing. Talk to him about it and how he is feeling about it.

Praise and Encouragement

Praise and encouragement are forms of positive attention that are easy to give and will motivate young children to behave. The line between praise and encouragement can be rather blurred but praise tends to concentrate on success and can be hard to live up to, for example "Wonderful boy!"

On the other hand, encouragement is sincere and does not exaggerate, for example you can say, "Oh, I see you have put some of your toys away today. That's helpful." While a little praise will not do any harm, encouragement appears to work better. Both work best when they are sincere and given frequently (but not all the time) and generously. So rather than saying "Good boy", say "Well done. You are working really hard at that."

Building Self-esteem and Encouraging Independence

Parents are sometimes reluctant to use these forms of positive attention as they feel it will make a child proud and, particularly with regard to praise, that the child will get hooked on it.

In reality, these forms of positive attention help to build self-esteem and if you use encouragement rather than praise, noticing effort and progress rather than just achievement, you will be encouraging independence.

Showing your child that you expect him to behave well can be a positive self-fulfilling prophecy. The reverse is also true, so it is best not to remind him of past misdemeanours which can have the effect of putting ideas in his head.

Extrinsic Rewards and Their Long-term Effects

Extrinsic rewards are things that are given to children as a reward for good behaviour, like stickers, toys or a food treat. Some parents and teachers use star charts or put marbles in a jar, adding a marble for good behaviour and taking one out for unwanted behaviour. A full jar means the child gets a desired toy or treat. Such methods work well in the short term or for particular targets parents want their child to achieve, like a dry bed at night.

However, in the long term, children can get hooked on getting a reward for everything they do or will do work only when there is a treat at the end of it all. It is better for children to be intrinsically motivated, that is to do something like learning for the satisfaction it gives.

Praise and attention are often just as effective as extrinsic rewards.

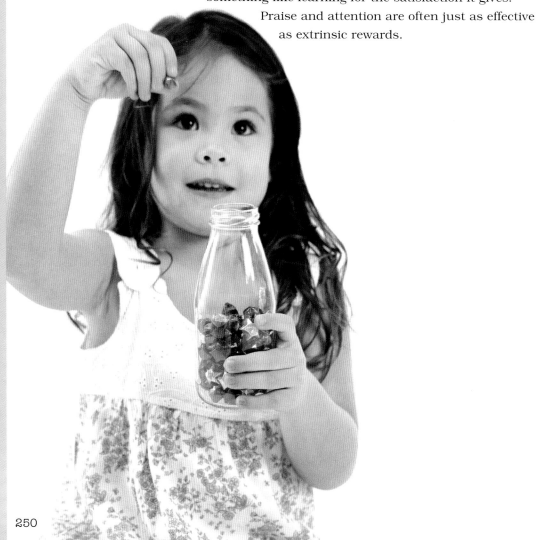

Overdoing Discipline and Under Disciplining

Learning to behave appropriately is a gradual process that is linked to your child's development in other areas, particularly his ability to think and use language. Your young child typically sees the world from his point of view—referred to as being egocentric—and so the 2-year-old with no concept of ownership may snatch toys. Such behaviour would not be acceptable from a 4-year-old. Age, however, is not the only measure to go by. Children vary in their development and an older child with learning difficulties or developmental delay may act like a much younger child, having tantrums or being aggressive.

Overdoing discipline can be harmful as it may stop some forms of poor behaviour but produce others. Children may become timid, withdrawn and fearful or conversely rebel and become anti-social, doing things like biting, stealing, being aggressive and having temper tantrums. The child may feel miserable because it seems he cannot do anything right and may doubt his parents love him.

Expectations that are too high may make the child feel like a failure and lead to constant nagging on the part of the parent.

If expectations are too low, the child may not learn appropriate behaviour for his age and may become greedy, selfish, rude, disobedient and uncooperative, making it difficult for the child to socialise. The child may also feel insecure because no limits are placed on his behaviour and be accident-prone as he is not aware of dangers.

Some Important Dos and Don'ts of Disciplining

* Do be consistent and act as a good role model—mixed messages will confuse your child.

* Do find out if the child care centre your child goes to follows a code of behaviour you are happy with.

* Do catch your child being good—noticing good behaviour encourages it.

* Do discipline your child as soon as possible after his misbehaviour.

* Do be aware that anger and other emotions are infectious.

* Do remember that labelling a child as shy, naughty or difficult tends to increase the risk of the unwanted behaviour.

* Do remember that being out of control is scary for a child. This can be when you get out of control or when your child gets out of control. Talk through the event and comfort your child when the anger has passed.

* Don't worry if you feel you have failed—persevere and try a different approach the next time.

* Don't discipline your child in front of others.

To Cane or Not to Cane?

Some parents who experienced physical punishment when young feel they feared their parents and suffer from low self-esteem as a result of the harsh treatment they received and do not want to inflict the same treatment on their children. Others contend that what did them no harm will not harm their children, and that children need to "feel some pain to learn". You have the right to make these decisions and use physical punishment, provided it does not cause "grievous harm". Whatever your decision, be aware of the arguments against physical punishment.

Arguments against Physical Punishment

* Smacking or caning does not teach the child how to resolve conflicts peacefully or how to control his anger.

* The child may learn that violence works and use it on others, including his own children when he becomes a parent.

* The fear of being smacked can lead to the child lying about his actions.

* The parent may underestimate his own strength or anger and really hurt the child.

* The child may not always understand why he is being smacked.

* The parent may not be consistent about when he smacks the child so the child becomes confused about what behaviour leads to smacking.

Time Out

Time out is a discipline technique of removing your child from the situation where the misbehaviour is occurring. It is suitable for children aged 2 years and above, as they are old enough to understand the concepts of "waiting" and "being quiet". Explain to your child what the procedure is about and walk him through it the first few times.

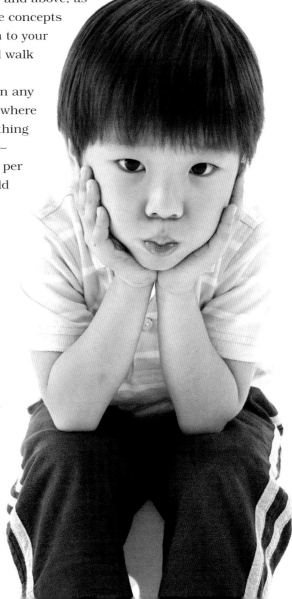

The time out place may be a chair in any room or a corner of the room, a place where he is isolated from others and has nothing to play with. The time needs to be age–appropriate: a good guide is 1 minute per year of life, so for a 3-year-old, it would be 3 minutes.

When you want your child to comply with a request, ask in a firm but pleasant tone. Give him time to do what you have asked and if he won't comply, make eye contact and say, "If you don't do what I've asked, you are going to have time out", and point to the chair. If he refuses to move, say in a firmer voice, "You did not do what I asked, so go and sit on the time out chair." Then take him by the hand and lead him there.

When the time out is over, explain to him what the appropriate behaviour is and then let him return to whatever he was doing.

Technology and Media

Modern homes are equipped with an array of electronic equipment. What is current changes quickly and many adults try to keep up with the latest in technology. Such interest in technology is easily picked up on by young children who are keen to explore all forms of it. What is the effect of technology and the media on your child's development and behaviour?

Children and Mobile Phones

The recent recommended age limit for the use of mobile phones, except in the case of an emergency, has been raised from below 7 to below 12 years of age. Adults are also being advised to restrict their own use of mobiles around children.

Mobile Phones

Mobile phones are an indispensable part of modern communication, making for instant accessibility. Toy makers produce versions for children but children are more fascinated with the real thing and are well aware of its uses.

Risks to Your Child

With a mobile phone being such an invasive and common feature of everyday life, you need to be aware of any possible risks to your child. While there is currently no data on mobile phone use and its risk of radiation/cancer in children, the possible health hazards make frightening reading: brain cancer, tumours leading to deafness, headaches, lack of concentration, memory loss, sleep disorders and even epilepsy. Until there is more concrete information about the risks to children, it is prudent to exercise caution and refrain from letting your child use your mobile phone too often.

TV

The recommended age for children to start watching TV is 2 years. If your child watches TV, here are some important points to be aware of.

Time Spent Watching TV

It is recommended that preschoolers watch no more than one to two hours of informative/quality programmes a day. Teach your child that programmes are for occasional entertainment rather than constant companionship.

Programme Selection

A review of TV watching and programmes conducted in the United States suggests that it is not how long children spend watching TV but what programmes they watch. They distinguished between children's programmes that were informative, like *Barney* and *Sesame Street*, and those that were purely entertainment.

Where children watched informative programmes, they were as likely to spend time on other educational-type activities as children who did not watch TV. When children watched more entertainment-type programmes, they spent less time reading and doing other educational activities.

News Programmes

While news programmes may be informative, they are not recommended for children under the age of 5 as they expose children visually to wars, violent crimes and horrific disasters. At this tender age, children have little understanding of the context and are emotionally vulnerable. Children who watch such content tend to have greater fears and anxieties as they view the world to be a dangerous place. They may become fearful of going outside and have problems sleeping.

Educational Programmes

Here is a list of American TV programmes for children that support language/literacy and are available in some Asian countries.

- *64 Zoo Lane*
- *Barney and Friends*
- *Jack's Big Music Show*
- *Oobi*
- *Oswald*
- *Pinky Dinky Doo*
- *Sesame Street*
- *The Upside Down Show*
- *Wilbur*
- *WordWorld*

Playhouse Disney learning goals are available from http://tv.disney.go.com/playhouse/grownups/aboutus.html

Source: *Young Children*, March 2009

Cartoons

What is the impact of violent cartoons on a child's behaviour? Children between the ages of 2 and 3 appear to find cartoons difficult to understand and lose concentration, so they may be immune to the messages.

For older preschoolers, the fact that the characters are animated rather than real and the context is obviously comic helps them to understand that it is not real life. Provided the child has developed the ability to distinguish between right and wrong, fantasy and reality, it seems unlikely that they will perpetrate violent acts in real life as a result of watching cartoons. However, children can get hooked on them, wanting to see the same cartoon repeatedly and become difficult to manage or engage.

Other Programmes

Seeing violent programmes where the characters are real people rather than cartoon characters has a greater negative impact on behaviour. Watching violent programmes is a significant factor in children either becoming victims of bullying or becoming aggressive themselves as they can either over-sensitise or desensitise children. Witnessing violence first hand at home or in the community has the greatest impact.

Some are quick to point out that violence has always been a part of children's lives and experiences—in nursery rhymes, myths, legends and stories, and in families and communities—and that 'playing' with violence in games and cartoons is one way children can make sense of it and possibly gain some control over it. However, violent images are now much more likely to intrude into homes and when children have an unhealthy liking for programmes with violent content, there is the need to talk to them about this and examine the family's viewing habits.

TV and Inattention in Children

The essence of TV is the moving screen and this in itself may contribute to inattention. The rapidly shifting images are thought to condition the brain to expect a higher level of stimulation than it encounters in normal everyday life, so normal activities lead to boredom and consequently inattention.

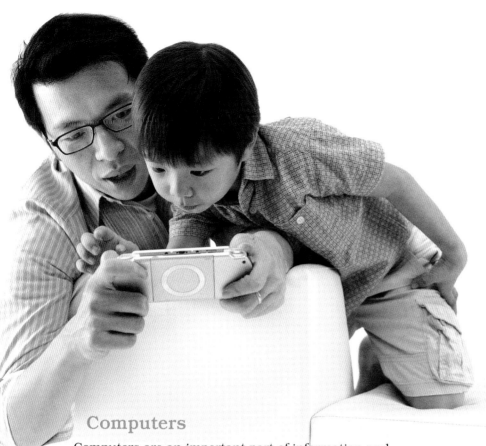

Computers

Computers are an important part of information and communication technology and are increasingly available in homes. As they are a part of twenty-first century living, your child needs to be exposed to them. To begin with, he can be introduced to other machines before or alongside computers, including gadgets like key finders, torches, digital clocks, timers, alarms and birthday cards that play tunes when opened.

Programmable toys like Roamers (educational robots that can be used for maths and language activities) as well as remote control cars show your child that he can control things by his thoughts and actions and are an alternative to computers.

Despite the necessity for computers, excessive use of the computer can be detrimental and:

✳ Cause eye strain.

✳ Lead to repetitive injuries.

✳ Restrict time for other more social, physical and outdoor activities, leading to obesity.

✳ Limit the opportunities to exercise creativity and imagination.

As computer use is largely a solitary activity, be aware that it may contribute towards your child becoming socially isolated and affect his language development.

Programme/Game Selection

As with TV, the type of programme or game that your child spends his time on needs to be considered. If there is a need to practise a skill, working on the computer may be more motivating than using pencil and paper, especially for boys, and might encourage the child to stay at the task longer.

Software that is developmentally appropriate can stimulate creativity, increase knowledge and contribute to developing your child's vocabulary. Similarly, games and drawing programmes can be educational and stimulate your child's critical thinking, creative problem solving and exploratory play.

Benefits of Computer Usage

Recent research has shown that there is a trend towards intellectual benefits as children are actively involved and in control when using the computer. Where adults or other children are on hand to give assistance or encourage discussion, the benefits increase.

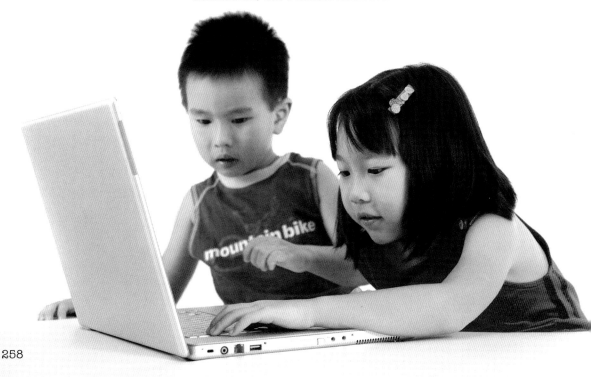

* There is no evidence from research that computer use enhances language but many programmes give children good exposure to language.

* Some software packages help children to learn about writing by scribing for them.

* For older preschoolers, using the computer in pairs can encourage interaction, learning from each other, sharing and turn-taking.

Controlling Your Child's Use of Media

Setting Limits on Usage

While technology is undoubtedly entertaining and informative for all the family, there needs to be control and limits on its use. Going to the computer/TV to be entertained should not become a default activity for your child. Train him to entertain himself. Play the role of both watch dog and guide to ensure that your child learns to control his behaviour and that he is learning the right things from what he watches.

Research has shown that when the TV is on all or most of the time, regardless of whether anyone is watching it or not, children have shorter attention spans, interact less with adults and are slower to learn to read.

Placing the Computer/TV in Common Areas

It is easier to monitor the usage of the computer and TV if they are kept in areas of the home shared by all family members and not in a bedroom. Research has shown that where parents allow computers/TV in the bedroom, children watch more and are more likely to be obese—the likelihood increasing with every extra hour they watch.

Asking for Permission

Maintain control of the TV remote and teach your child to ask before turning on the TV. Like chocolate, children can have too much of a good thing.

Time Limit or Programme Limit

Setting limits can involve imposing a time limit or setting a limit on the number of programmes a child can watch. Where parents set time limits, the child tends to watch less. Where parents set programme limits, the child tends to watch more. Talk to your child about the need to set limits so that he knows that you do it because you care about him.

Additional Tips on the Use of Media

✳ Take charge of the media in your home. Your child needs as much help, if not more, in controlling this area of his behaviour. He needs to learn to live in the real world and not retreat into a virtual world.

✳ Keep yourself informed about good programmes and software for children that conveys positive images about their gender and ethnicity, and is educational as well as engaging. Remember that your child will only benefit from using or watching what is developmentally appropriate.

✳ Allow for some relaxation and fun watching.

✳ Use the computer as a learning tool with your preschooler but not to the exclusion of other more interactive and tried and tested ways of learning, like sharing picture books, playing games, singing and saying rhymes together.

✳ Watch TV or use the computer together with your child as much as possible. Children benefit more when adults are involved and discussion ensues.

✳ Keep yourself informed about safe surfing. Use groups like Parents Advisory Group for the Internet, Singapore (PAGI) to keep you up-to-date.

✳ Don't ignore warning signals like your child's need to be constantly entertained by watching TV.

✳ Don't use the TV as a regular baby sitter and make sure your child care centre does not do this as well. Teachers should watch alongside the children and already have previewed the content.

ADVERTISING AND ITS EFFECTS ON CHILDREN

You may question the relevance of considering the role of advertising when talking about preschoolers. Unfortunately, children as young as 2 can be influenced by it, through the TV and other screen-based media. There is growing concern that children are being increasingly targeted at ages when they are easily brainwashed because they lack the critical ability to evaluate marketing tactics.

Toys linked to the programmes children watch or the computer games they play, often labelled with the magic word "educational", are advertised in such a way that children pester parents to buy them as their friends have them. Peer pressure starts early too! Be wary about rushing out to purchase things that your child wants without checking to see if they are really worthwhile.

Educationists have always contended that the best toys for exercising a child's creativity and imagination are often the simplest: a cardboard box, a 'den' under a table, a box of old clothes to dress up in and crayons and paper, but these make little if any money, and in the world of advertising, children are now considered to be big business.

Increasingly, children are being introduced to the competitive world of brands. Studies have found that preschoolers between the ages of 2 and 5 can influence their parents over the brands of food and snacks they buy and, by the age of 3, can ask for brands by name. Be aware of marketing ploys and exert your influence over your child's thinking and behaviour while he is still a preschooler.

Some Dos and Don'ts

- ☐ Do be aware of advertising and marketing that target children.

- ☐ Do talk to your child about advertising and brands at a level he can understand.

- ☐ Don't give in to your child simply because he pesters you. Make a considered choice.

- ☐ Don't be consumed by brands yourself if you want to be a positive influence on your child.

Getting Ready for School

Early Education

Children develop at different rates. Some children mature earlier than others—physically, emotionally and intellectually. Although many parents enrol their children for preschool in the year they turn 4, not all children are mature and independent enough to start school. How can you tell if your child is ready to start preschool?

Is Your Child Ready?

Age is only one of the factors to consider when deciding if your child is ready for nursery school. Having simple physical skills such as being able to fasten buttons or catch a ball, and simple language skills such as communicating his needs and describing his feelings, will indicate if your child is able to cope in nursery school. It is therefore important that you judge your child's capabilities as a whole.

Here are some of the things that he should be able to do:

* Know his own name.

* Follow simple instructions.

* Dress himself.

* Feed himself.

* Use the toilet.

* Wash his face and hands.

* Share toys and take turns without getting upset.

* Hold pencils and crayons to scribble or write.

* Cut and paste.

If he is still not ready, it will be more beneficial if you let him stay home for one more year to develop and become more independent. In fact, some studies have shown that the older a child is when starting nursery school, the greater his readiness.

Your child is ready for preschool when he is able to:

* Play happily with other children.

* Make friends.

* Cope with new challenges.

* Ask for help when necessary.

* Be able to control his behaviour.

* Take some responsibility for his own belongings.

* Respect the belongings of others.

* Sit still for extended periods to listen to stories and work on his drawing or colouring activities.

Boys Versus Girls

There is a popular view that boys should start preschool a year later than girls. This is because compared to girls, some boys are not observed to be developmentally ready for school. Because of their immaturity, 4- and 5-year-old boys are seen to be unable to use their fingers to manage tasks such as cutting, colouring and drawing, and their attention spans are more limited than those of girls of the same age. Starting nursery school before they have the necessary hand and eye coordination to manage such tasks may account for some boys' unhappiness about school and the difficulties they have coping in the early school years. However, once they reach the age of 7 or 8, most boys will have matured sufficiently to enable them to match the abilities of girls when doing such tasks.

All this suggests that if the nursery school provides a play-based environment where boys are encouraged to thrive rather than focusing on what they cannot do, and where their achievements are valued, their self-confidence will improve and outweigh any deficits in their development compared to girls.

Prepare Your Child

Be enthusiastic as you talk to your child about going to school. If he senses anxiety in your voice, mannerisms or gestures, he will not be reassured and may become anxious himself.

* Tell him about the fun things that can happen at school, such as meeting new friends, playing with new toys, wearing a smart new uniform and, for some, going to school on the school bus.

* Borrow books from the library and read to your child about starting school.

* Familiarise your child with other people and their children, perhaps by going together to a mother and toddler group or by inviting other parents and their children to your home on a few occasions.

* Encourage your child to be independent by praising him for tasks accomplished unaided such as washing and bathing, using the toilet, dressing and fastening clothing, answering the telephone or making telephone calls. You can do this through pretend play.

* Familiarise your child with the school from the outside, by driving or walking past while you talk encouragingly about what a wonderful time he will have, just as a sibling or you yourself did when first starting nursery school.

* Make a point to visit the school with your child and ask to see your child's classroom and note the names of the principal, class teacher and assistants as well as the administrative staff. Knowing this information will reinforce your and your child's eagerness to start school.

* Meet and talk with the principal and class teacher. This building of relationships before school starts will help to ease the settling-in period.

As the day for starting school gets closer, it will be exciting for your child to wear his school uniform at home and to be encouraged to show it to other family members who may comment on how clever and grown-up your child has become. This will help boost your child's confidence.

The First Day at School

It is natural for your child, and you, to feel a mixture of anxiety, euphoria and apprehension as he takes this first major step in his life. On the first day, it is best to stay with your child until he feels comfortable and absorbed in an activity before you leave.

Reassure your child that you will return soon to take him home. Teachers have their ways of distracting new children and most children will stop crying after a while and join in the activities. However, it is important to keep your promise and return on time at the end of the school session or you will lose the trust you have painstakingly built up to the big day.

Understand School Requirements and Regulations

Check the school newsletters and bulletin boards for any information that will help your child during the early settling-in period. Find out about any essential requirements and regulations such as those for administering medication, being absent from school and wearing jewellery or other accessories.

Adjusting to the School Environment

It is quite normal for your child to be unhappy about returning to school after the initial enthusiasm has worn off. When this happens, you will have to continue with your enthusiastic and reinforcing support. It is difficult for young children to realise and understand that once they have started nursery school, they are in it for the long haul.

Since this new routine is not part of the home environment where parents or caregivers provide undivided and loving attention, it is difficult for young children to have to share the teacher's attention with other children on top of all the new rules and regulations that they are subjected to at

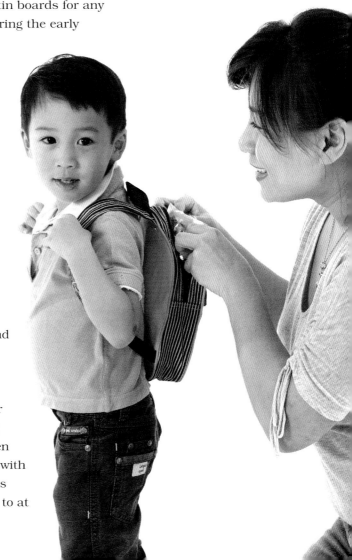

school. All these can be overwhelming and your child may be disillusioned by school. He may act up at home, wet his bed or have difficulty sleeping.

Keep Your Child's Teacher Informed

Let your child's teacher know of any difficulties your child may be experiencing and she will be able to advise and support your child through any difficult periods.

It is important though that your child continues to attend school during this time otherwise the settling-in process will have to be repeated and may take much longer a second time around. However, as school routines become more familiar and he begins to build new relationships with adults and other children, he will eventually settle down.

Listen to Your Child

Listen to your child's comments on the day's activities with interest and enthusiasm. Refrain from asking too many questions; rather, wait for your child to tell you in his own time. While all this is happening, don't expect too much from the settling-in process. Don't be affected by what other parents tell you and don't try to compare your child's progress with that of other children. Children cope with new events and experiences in different ways and at different rates. Adjusting to these changes positively will take time and will demand patience from both parents and teachers.

Get to Know Your Child's Teachers

It is important to maintain contact with teachers and administrators in your child's preschool. Your child's teacher is the person your child will grow attached to and there needs to be a basic sense of trust among you: the teacher, you and your child.

Talk to the teacher about your child's progress on a regular basis. Share your doubts and fears as well as your high points with the teacher. Parents and teachers working together go a long way in determining the quality of the settling-in process.

CHOOSING A PRESCHOOL

Preschools in Singapore comprise child care centres and kindergartens. The Ministry of Education (MOE) monitors the kindergartens whilst the Ministry of Community Development, Youth and Sports (MCYS) licenses child care centres. Nursery schools/classes are found in both kindergartens and child care centres. There are some things that you may want to find out when choosing a preschool for your child. These include:

- ☐ The school's aims and philosophy.

- ☐ The curriculum.

- ☐ The teaching strategy.

- ☐ Activities provided at the school.

- ☐ The physical environment—the indoor and outdoor spaces—are they well ventilated, safe, etc.

- ☐ The kind of equipment and other resources available.

- ☐ The interaction between children and adults at the school.

- ☐ How the children's performance and progress are monitored and evaluated.

It is a good idea to visit a few centres and talk to the teachers and other parents. Choose the school where you feel most at ease and where you think your child will be safe and happy.

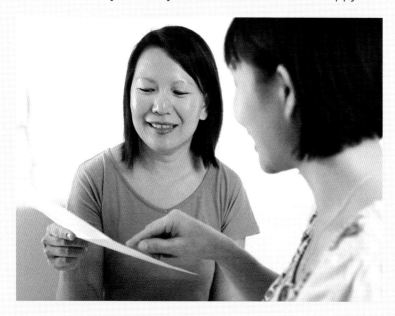

CHILD CARE CENTRES
Programmes in Child Care Centres
Infant Care
For children aged 2 to 18 months

Child Care
For children above 18 months to below 7 years

Number of Hours Per Week
These can be half- or full-day, flexible-care (12, 24, 36 and 48 hours per week) and emergency care.

Hours of Operation
Mondays to Fridays from 7:00 am to 7:00 pm
Saturdays from 7:00 am to 2:00 pm

Staff-Child Ratios in Child Care Centres

2 months to 18 months	1 teacher to 5 children
Above 18 months to 30 months	1 teacher to 8 children
Above 30 months to 3 years	1 teacher to 12 children
Above 3 years to 4 years	1 teacher to 15 children
Above 4 years to below 7 years	1 teacher to 25 children

These centres are assessed for licensing purposes according to the physical environment, safety, health, hygiene and nutrition, staff training/qualifications and staffing requirements, the programme and curriculum, and administration.

Further information on child care centres, and especially how to select a suitable centre for your child, can be obtained from MCYS.

MCYS, Child Care Division
510 Thomson Road
#13-00 SLF Building
Singapore 298135
Telephone: (65) 6258 5812
Email: mcys_child_care_link@mcys.gov.sg
Website: www.childcarelink.gov.sg

KINDERGARTENS
Programmes in Kindergartens

Kindergarten programmes are for children between the ages of 3 and 6 years of age and comprise Nursery (N1 and N2), Kindergarten 1 (K1) and Kindergarten 2 (K2) classes. Each individual kindergarten has its own registration procedures, usually starting from March each year for admission in January of the following year. Further information about kindergartens can be obtained from the MOE website (www. moe.gov.sg/education/preschool).

Some key points about the selection of appropriate kindergartens for your child that come from this website are mentioned here for reference:

☐ Location. On the Pre-school Education page, click on "Finding a Kindergarten". This will enable you to look for the specific locations of kindergartens (by postal code).

☐ Qualifications of teachers and principals.

☐ The kindergarten programme. Read more about this by downloading the article "A Framework for a Kindergarten Curriculum in Singapore" from the MOE website. Talk to the kindergarten's principal for more information.

☐ Class sizes. Nursery classes are recommended to have one teacher and one teacher aide to 15 children; K1 classes should have a maximum of one teacher to 20 children; K2 classes should have a maximum of one teacher to 25 children.

In order to select the most appropriate setting for your child, it is advisable to consult these websites or make visits to MCYS and MOE. Thereafter, visit a selection of settings to check which setting best matches your child's needs. You could also talk to other parents and seek their advice.

If your child starts school with positive self-esteem and has the ability to control and express his feelings in socially acceptable ways and respond agreeably to others using well-developed social skills, he will not only be more likely to succeed as a learner at school but will also be better equipped to get along with his peers.

Basic Social Skills

Below are the five basic social skills that your child needs for school. He should be able to:

* Carry on a conversation (which involves listening and waiting for his turn to speak).

* Take turns.

* Correctly interpret the action of others.

* Share.

* Come up with good solutions to conflicts.

Carry On a Conversation and Take Turns

Carrying on a conversation involves a child patiently waiting for his turn before speaking. Use puppets to let your child practise this skill. For example:

Puppet A: Good morning, good morning and how are you?
Puppet B: Good morning, good morning, I'm very well thank you.

Correctly Interpret the Action of Others

Interpreting the actions of others is not easy. A less socially competent child will often misread the actions of others and this can cause conflicts. For example, Peter sticks out his tongue to show Jim that it is orange after drinking orange juice. A less socially competent child might come to the wrong conclusion that Peter is being rude to him and hit him.

The child who is socially competent is good at observing and watching others at play and assessing their behaviour.

He is therefore able to anticipate what he needs to do in certain situations.

Kim, 5 years old

Kim wanted to join the group of children at the puppet theatre who were improvising their own play with puppets. She watched them for a while and then offered to help close the curtain at the end of the performance. One of the boys refused her offer and said it was his job to close the curtain. Kim then asked if she could help the children pack the puppets back into their boxes, an offer that no one rejected!

Kim was unruffled by the boy rejecting her offer to close the curtain and immediately came up with another idea. The socially competent child does not get too upset when he fails to get what he wants.

Share

Sharing is one of the most difficult social skills for a child to acquire as it involves taking on the view of another, which developmentally is a fairly advanced task. A toddler therefore finds it difficult to share, but by about the age of 4, he will be ready to do this. Here is an example to help you find out how much your child understands about sharing.

Jenny, 4 years old

Jenny is having a tea party. She has invited her daddy and her favourite stuffed toy, Mr Bear. "Mummy has made some cakes," Daddy says, and places a plate containing four cakes on the table. "Can you help me share them out between us?" he asks. He then guides Jenny in placing one cake at a time on each plate. He then directs Jenny's attention to the one remaining cake and asks Jenny, "What shall we do with the cake that is left over?"

Jenny could respond in a number of ways to her father's question. Depending on how she answers shows us the level of reasoning she is using to solve this problem. She could suggest:

* Taking it for herself.

* Dividing it in two—half for her and half for her father.

* Splitting it three ways so Mr Bear can have some too.

* Giving it to Mummy (who is not present at the party).

You can play out different scenarios to help your child develop social skills needed in different situations involving sharing. Doing jigsaw puzzles, for example, will help your child learn that he has to contribute his pieces to others so the puzzle can be completed successfully.

Come Up with Good Solutions to Conflicts

If your child argues even with his friends, it is usually because he does not want to share something. Help him learn how to share by guiding him to negotiate and take turns to reach a happy compromise. It is important to help your child to learn to be assertive to get what he wants while controlling his negative feelings.

The child who has been rewarded for pro-social behaviour, like sharing and helping at home, with parents modelling such behaviour for him tends to:

* Be more helpful than other children.

* Play more cooperatively and harmoniously with other children.

* Be able to follow the teacher's instructions.

* Be able to empathise with and comfort other children.

* Show affection and care.

* Be honest and fair.

* Respect the property of others.

Making Friends

There is a lot of give and take involved in friendships. It is mutual, reciprocal play that cements friendships among children between the ages of 4 and 7. This is the stage where your child will indulge in a lot of fantasy play, switching roles with friends, giving instructions and assuming leadership roles.

The first stable friendships begin to emerge at this stage with your child choosing friends of the same sex. He will seek out his new friends to play with and may get upset if they are absent from school.

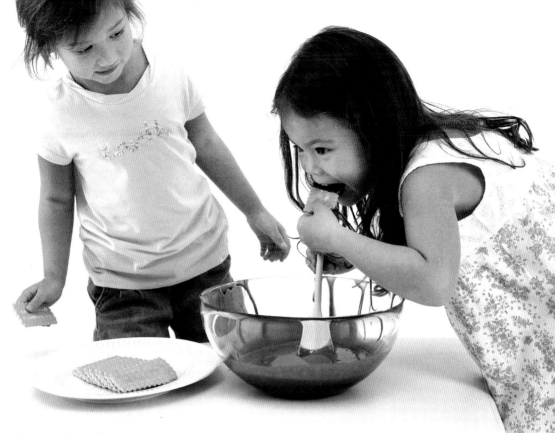

Making Friends Isn't Easy!

Don't assume that your child will easily make friends. The initial, and probably the most difficult, skill that your child needs is to gain entry into a group.

Developing Access Strategies

Gaining entry into a group often presents problems for children who may unwittingly 'barge' into an ongoing group activity thinking they will be immediately accepted. Children need to develop access strategies to break the ice with others. See the earlier example of Kim (page 271).

The child who is willing to wait and watch has been likened to a tiger encircling its prey waiting for the right opportunity to strike. He then follows up with a side by side strategy, which involves him imitating what the other children are doing.

For example, on an outing to the playground, Lee's father sees a group of children playing in the sandpit and says, "Lee, do you want to join in? Look at what they are doing. They are pouring sand in and out of pots. There's no need to ask them if you can join in, just do the same as them."

As suggested in this example, it is better to just join in and not ask permission in case the other children say "No!". Rejection might damage Lee's confidence to join in group play in the future. A more confident child might, like Kim, use other strategies like inviting himself into a group or initiating a group activity and then inviting others to join in!

The Popular Child

The popular child is good at using such access strategies and acting in positive ways which then attract other children to be his friends. Such a child will take the initiative to say nice things, for example, "I like you" or offer comfort and help "Let me carry that book for you" or be willing to share something "Have one of my cakes."

Characteristics of the Popular Child

* Cooperates with others.

* Waits his turn.

* Willingly shares his things.

* Is fair to all.

* Is tactful and sensitive to the feelings of others.

* Knows how to bargain and negotiate with his peers.

* Is able to resolve conflicts without being aggressive or breaking rules and only appeals to the teacher for help when all else has failed.

The Unpopular Child

The child who finds it difficult to make friends runs the risk of being labelled as "unpopular". This child is usually over-demanding, aggressive or shy.

The Over-demanding Child

The over-demanding child is invariably the only child in the family and/or has been the centre of attention at home. He:

* Is used to getting his own way.

* Has not learnt how to wait and take turns.

* Has had his needs met immediately at home.

* Has had his good behaviour purchased rather than earned.

* Feels insecure in the social setting of the school as he does not have the family to protect him.

* Appears ill at ease with other children.

Helping the Over-demanding Child

The over-demanding child needs sensitive and sustained support to become involved initially in parallel play with other children before graduating to group activities that require cooperation and sharing, such as completing simple jigsaw puzzles or contributing to an art collage.

He may try to buy friends by offering his peers the chance to play with the status possessions he owns, like the latest toy on the market. This child needs to understand that controlling friends in this way will not help him develop long-term quality relationships. He needs to be guided in his social interactions to demonstrate that it is his ideas and willingness to go with the flow of the group activity that other children will value, not what material objects he can entice them with in order to get them to be friends with him.

The Aggressive Child

The aggressive child is also unpopular at school because:

* He is unable to control his feelings or behaviour and runs the risk of being rejected by his peers.

* He does not have the necessary language to say what he wants and uses proactive aggression to get what he wants, such as snatching things from another child.

* He reacts aggressively when provoked or frustrated and lashes out at others in the heat of the moment with the deliberate intention of hurting someone.

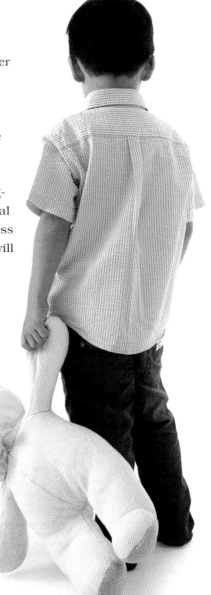

Helping the Aggressive Child

The goal of any intervention to help the aggressive child is to help him become more socially acceptable and to learn how to become assertive without being aggressive. Research has revealed that aggressive preschoolers who are rejected by their peers experience higher levels of stress than children whose behaviour is more socially acceptable. Parents should try to:

* Build up the child's confidence to make him feel good about himself.

* Praise him when he uses social skills that are acceptable.

* Help him filter some of the frustration he feels about not being in control of the situation.

* Provide him with activities (closely monitored) that help him vent his anger. For example, dough play, using musical instruments and climbing during outdoor play as well as do more calming activities like sand play.

The Shy Child

Should parents worry if their child is shy? Will he be at risk of being rejected by his peers and vulnerable to teasing and bullying? The shy child does run the risk of being rejected by his peers. He also finds it awkward to be part of the group in certain situations. He therefore needs to be monitored closely and paired with a more empathetic and socially mature child who can be on hand to ease him into larger social circles at school.

How You Can Help

There is often a certain amount of pain involved in early childhood relationships, but it is all part of learning. You might feel helpless and anxious when your child's life becomes more complicated and friendships shift from day to day, but what your child needs is for you to support him when he turns to you in both happy and sad times. Here's how you can support your child.

* Don't be over-anxious. Most children will bounce back from rejections and the inevitable betrayals involved in early friendships.

* Help your child develop empathy and reciprocity by being a good model. Ask him to hug you when you are upset and demonstrate the give-and-take involved in loving relationships.

* Share stories that have been especially crafted to support children in their efforts to develop pro-social behaviour. A short bibliotherapy is provided under Resources (pages 344–345).

* Find out about your child's social status. If you suspect that he is having social problems at school, talk with his teacher to find out if he is behaving in ways which are irritating to others, then work out how you can help.

* Arrange a variety of group friendship opportunities. Plan play-dates with other children from the preschool. If your child seems isolated at school, you might need to find another social circle for him to find a friend, such as around your neighbourhood or at a swimming class.

* Make your child accountable for his behaviour at school. You need to confront your child if you find out he has been indulging in unacceptable behaviour. For example, teasing or bullying. Tell him straight out that you will not stand for it because you find it a mean way to behave.

* Don't be influenced by what other parents say. Parents never get accurate information about the social lives their children lead at school. It is advisable not to listen to the gossip and comparisons other parents indulge in at the school gates.

* Listen to your child. Spend time letting your child tell you about his problems and don't overreact by trying to help him find solutions for every problem.

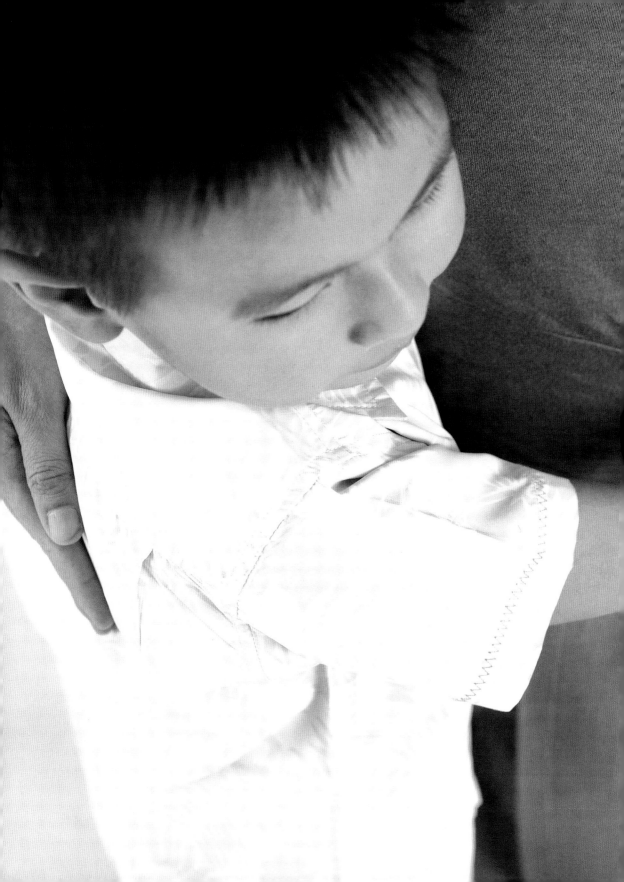

The Child with Special Needs

While all children need encouragement and support as they move along the path of learning, some children need more time and help than others. They may be considered to have special needs and be at risk of not doing well at school.

Contributor:
Asst Prof Linda Gan

Developmental Disorders

This section covers the developmental disorders that have received the most attention over the past 10 years because of the observations of teachers and an ever-increasing amount of knowledge provided by the medical profession. They are attention deficit hyperactivity disorder (ADHD), dyslexia and autism spectrum disorder (ASD).

The Preschool Years

According to research, these disorders affect more boys than girls. The characteristic behaviour of these disorders usually appears during the preschool years. The information in this chapter will help parents to be alert to the needs of their child and to seek appropriate advice or medical help.

Attention Deficit Hyperactivity Disorder (ADHD)

Lee, 3 years old

Lee is an unusually active and busy 3-year-old. His mother likens him to a bullet being fired from a gun! He is forever dashing around and never seems to sit still in one place for more than a few minutes. Even when playing, he darts from one activity to another. His new Lego set lies scattered in pieces around the floor... he gets easily bored and does not have the patience to put together more than a few blocks at a time before getting frustrated and bursting into tears if others try to help him. His latest adventure at home was throwing crayons into the washing machine before his mother could stop him and ruining all his father's shirts. At his small playgroup, he is very demanding and noisy and is unpopular with the other children as he is constantly interfering in their play. His parents confess he drains all energy from them as they are constantly on the go to help protect him and others from his wild ways.

Lee is just one of an increasing number of 3- to 5-year-olds who display such behaviour and have been diagnosed with ADHD. Parents often put such hyperactive behaviour down to the endless energy 3-year-olds are known to possess, especially boys! But as the child gets older and moves into the more structured environment of preschool, teachers will inevitably start to communicate their concern to parents over their child's tendency to act first and think later, the constant squirming, fidgeting, running and jumping, and possibly his physical and social clumsiness. These children also often have trouble with gross and fine motor skills and, as a result, are accident-prone. This clumsiness usually extends to social relationships with other children, who often exclude ADHD children because of their impulsive and intrusive behaviour.

It is tempting for parents to jump to the conclusion that their hyperactive toddler is suffering from ADHD. However, they first need to observe their child over a protracted period of time before consulting a doctor who can refer them for a professional diagnosis.

The young child who is suspected of having ADHD will usually:

* Have difficulty sitting still and always be on the go.

* Have a very short attention span.

* Be easily distracted by environmental sights and sounds.

* Have difficulty playing quietly.

* Interrupt or interfere with what others are doing.

* Appear unable to listen when spoken to.

* Appear unable to follow through on instructions and fail to complete tasks.

* Experience great difficulty in getting organised and following routines.

Causes of ADHD

ADHD is known to be caused by insufficient neurochemicals which impair the child's ability to control attention and inhibition. These characteristics are more pronounced when the child with ADHD enters a more structured learning environment, which makes demands on him to sit still and listen for long periods of time.

In Asian cultures, a lot of stress is laid on discipline and, in general, the hyperactive child is not tolerated. Many will find it hard to be patient with such a naughty child who continues to exhibit such behaviour throughout childhood and adolescence. Many symptoms, particularly hyperactivity, diminish in early adulthood, but impulsivity and inattention problems remain with up to 50 percent of ADHD individuals throughout their adult life.

Once diagnosed, early intervention, mainly by teachers and educational psychologists, is crucial to help the child with ADHD to fit in to more formal learning environments as well as build up his self-confidence and social skills to overcome other challenges that might present themselves as he gets older. If the child's behaviour warrants more intensive intervention, then a multi-modal approach will probably be suggested to the parents, which might involve medication, family counselling and a behaviour management programme at home and at school.

Suggestions for Parents

* Establish the same routine every day from wake-up time to bedtime. If the schedule needs to be changed, make it as far in advance as possible.

* Have a place for everything and keep everything in place (including clothes, books, toys, etc).

✽ Make rules the child can understand and follow. Be consistent about applying them and if followed, give small rewards. The child with ADHD often expects criticism so be constantly on the lookout for good behaviour and praise it!

✽ Provide a lot of free play to keep the child active and busy. Be there to support him and keep him at the task, giving him regular breaks during activities that demand more attention. The younger the child, the more frequent the breaks. (For example, 5-minute intervals for 3-year-olds.)

✽ Find out what holds the child's interest and build on this.

✽ Avoid long explanations—show rather than tell.

✽ For tasks needing more attention, create an area that is free from distractions.

Learning to Cope

It is easier said than done to advise parents with a child suffering from ADHD to stay calm as it is extremely frustrating to have to constantly check their active and impulsive behaviour. It is important though for parents to avoid outright confrontation with their child and not to be scared to admit that on certain days, they are not coping well and need others to step in and take over.

It is also very important to find comfort and support from other parents who have children with ADHD. The Society for the Promotion of ADHD Research and Knowledge (SPARK) holds a parent support group meeting on the first Saturday of every month at the Health Promotion Board Building near Singapore General Hospital. This is a time where parents can discuss experiences and the strategies they use to help them and their children cope with this disorder.

Dyslexia

Dyslexia means "word blindness" and it is a long-term problem that affects normal, intelligent people who, despite the best attempts by skilled teachers to instruct them, still have difficulty reading.

Ben, 5 years old

Ben is an intelligent, curious 5-year-old with a vivid imagination. He loves painting and drawing and spends a lot of time creating objects out of paper and clay. He enjoys being read to but becomes very irritable when asked to help with reading a book, preferring instead to look at and comment on the illustrations. In fact, he has told his parents that the black squiggles (words) seem to jump all over the place on the page and make him feel giddy. He has been attending a phonics enrichment programme for the past few months but finds it very stressful and has made no progress at all. He becomes equally frustrated when he has to write his name. The other children in his class have started to tease him about this and he is strongly resisting going to school because he says they call him "Dumbo".

It is estimated that 3 to 5 percent of Singaporeans may be dyslexic. Like Ben, they are very competent at expressing themselves verbally but have great difficulty putting their ideas down on paper. They repeatedly reverse consonants like "b", "d" and "p", and have problems with literacy activities, except speaking. They make up for their deficiency in reading and writing by thinking in pictures rather than words and prefer hands-on activities where they can give life to their ideas in more artistic activities.

Causes of Dyslexia

Researchers generally agree that the cause of dyslexia is neurological. Dyslexics have been found to suffer from some brain-based phonological deficit which stops them from breaking down words they hear or see written into their component sounds to help them read, spell and write.

Various factors complicate the identification and diagnosis of dyslexia. Firstly, claims that children as young as 2 or 3 can read are misleading. Most children learn to read when they are between 4½ and 7 years old. Parents are therefore cautioned not to overreact if their preschooler seems to be experiencing difficulties in learning to read and make the assumption that he is dyslexic. Furthermore, nearly all preschool children pass through the stage of reversing "b" or "d" or numbers like "2" and "9". They are essentially experimenting with letters and numbers and need guidance and practice to help them remember which direction these letters and numbers face.

Finally, reliable means to accurately assess why a child is struggling with learning how to read is crucial as it might be a direct consequence of external factors like poor preparation and poor teaching. Reading is a complex process and many preschool teachers might not be adequately trained to understand and effectively teach the skills involved.

The young child who is suspected of being dyslexic will usually:

* Have problems in reading, writing and spelling.

* Have phonological processing problems which prevent him from understanding that the words on paper are made up of the same number and patterns of sounds as the word being spoken.

* Constantly reverse consonants like "b", "d", "p" and "q" and numbers "2", "3", "4", "5", "7" and "9" when writing.

* Be very disorganised and find it difficult to remember a list of instructions—for example, what to take to school every day.

Suggestions for Parents

It is understandable for parents to panic if their child is experiencing problems with reading and writing as the education system in Singapore makes demands on children to be effectively biliterate in English and their own mother tongue. However, genuine dyslexia is unlikely to be detected until the child starts to fall behind in literacy activities at primary school. If parents take their preschool child too early for a diagnosis, it may not be accurate.

The Dyslexic Association of Singapore (DAS) provides assessment services and professional individual help for children they diagnose as dyslexic.

On a positive note, most children who experience reading problems are not developmentally dyslexic and will make sound progress if given correct instruction in reading. The advent of computer-assisted auditory training promises hope for those affected to overcome their disability.

Autism Spectrum Disorder (ASD)

Autism spectrum disorder (ASD) is a lifelong developmental disability. It includes the child with autism and Asperger syndrome. The characteristic features of autism typically appear before the age of 2½ years and the child is described as sitting on the other side of a mirror—able to observe what is going on in the world around him, but having little desire or inclination to be part of it. He typically experiences problems in social communication, social interaction and displays bizarre patterns of behaviour.

Siew Yee, 2½ years old

Siew Yee is engrossed in her daily routine of arranging all her toy phones around her and punching the buttons on each of them in turn. She is oblivious to everything going on around her until her mother inadvertently disturbs the perfect pattern of toys lying on the floor, which causes her to fly into a tantrum. She resists her mother's hugs to calm her down and howls in protest and wriggles furiously until her mother releases her. She then proceeds to return to punching the buttons on each of her toys as though nothing has happened, lost in her own private world, until she hears the introductory music to her favourite TV programme in the next room. Her mother finds her, 10 minutes later, sitting right on top of the TV set, wildly flapping her arms about, echoing the words of the programme's signature tune in a dull, monotonous tone.

Siew Lee's behaviour is in marked contrast to that of a normal 2½-year-old who would be enthusiastically exploring and playing with a variety of toys and objects, seeking comfort in her parents' hugs and kisses and using language to communicate her needs and desires to them and others around her.

The child suffering from ASD will:

* Indulge in self-stimulation by repeating stereotypical movements, like hand flapping, rocking and twirling around.

* Become obsessed with these actions which become cast in a set routine that cannot be interfered with.

* Be fascinated with certain stimuli, for example things that spin or rotate.

* Fly into uncontrollable tempers.

* Reject affection and bodily contact with others and avoid making eye contact with them.

* Imitate or echo the language he hears in a flat, monotonous tone.

* Be a social isolate, preferring to play alone.

* Exhibit very little variety and imagination in his play.

* Be unable to empathise with others.

* Indulge in social interaction only as a means to obtain something he wants or to talk solely about his interests.

* Have a limited sense of humour.

* Be rather clumsy as his gross and fine motor coordination skills are weak.

Causes of ASD

Recent research suggests ASD could be caused by biological factors like abnormal brain development, structure and neurochemistry. The majority of children diagnosed with this disorder are intellectually disabled with only 20 percent having average or above average intelligence. A minority may have advanced levels of ability in particular areas, like mathematics or art, which are known as savant skills. ASD can occur with other disorders like ADHD, so it is important for parents to have their child professionally diagnosed as soon as possible in order to ensure the child receives effective treatment.

Asperger Syndrome

The child with this milder form of autism may not be as severely delayed in his development and may be average or above average in intelligence. He is still impaired however in his communication, social and motor coordination skills, displays repetitive and stereotyped behaviour and insists on sticking to certain routines.

The child is able to attend mainstream pre- and primary schools in Singapore as part of the government's inclusion policy for children with special needs. Specialised staff are on hand to help the classroom teacher create an orderly structured learning environment in order to accommodate the child's need for strict routines and to advise him on handling other problems that might occur. For example, tolerating the child's behaviour and lack of social graces and skills. The child will invariably snatch things he wants rather than ask first and are apt to laugh at things that are not intended as jokes which makes him very unpopular with his peers, often resulting in him being bullied.

Suggestions for Parents

Delay in developing speech usually sets off the first alarm bell for parents to seek advice. When speech does start to appear, it is abnormal in terms of content and delivery. The child will echo what other people are saying to them in a flat, monotonous tone and usually use the third person "you" rather than using the personal pronoun "I". Parents will also be alerted very early on to the distressing realisation that their child seems oblivious to their overtures of love and affection, and seeks them out only when he needs something.

It is advisable to arrange for a referral as soon as possible to a professional educational psychologist for a diagnosis to be made. The Autism Resource Centre (ARC) offers a diagnostic service for children aged 4 and above and very comprehensive services for parents with children suffering from ASD. Once diagnosed, an early intervention programme can be drawn up to meet the child's individual needs. This will usually focus on educational and behaviour modification.

Parents with a child diagnosed with ASD will benefit from the support of other parents who have come to terms with the fact that their child is going to need their constant love and support throughout their lives. ARC and The Autism Association provides a source of help for parents.

Support for Parents

Many parents, especially fathers, go through a process of denial when their child is first suspected of having any of the disorders just discussed. This is an understandable reaction, but it is crucial for both parents to come together as soon as possible to work as partners to address the problems their child will face and to provide the emotional security and love he will need.

Most intervention programmes are designed for home and school use, and parents are usually the best people to motivate their child to complete the tasks set and to observe the progress being made in the informal and authentic context of the home.

Support for the Child with Special Needs

The child suffering from ADHD or dyslexia needs help to boost his self-esteem once he enters primary school, especially in an exam-orientated education system like Singapore's. Because exams generally involve reading and writing, the dyslexic child is immediately at a serious disadvantage as is the child with ADHD who, because of his short attention span, may rush through his exam papers without stopping to check his answers.

It is therefore very important for parents and teachers to help the child understand that it is the nature of his disability that is frustrating his chances of getting good grades. He needs to be reassured that he is not stupid and that it might take him longer to make the same progress as his peers in his overall learning journey. For him, it may take "a lot of slow to grow…"

Useful Contacts

Subsidised Venues for Diagnosis in Singapore

Child Guidance Clinic (CGC)

Health Promotion Board Building
3 Second Hospital Avenue, #03-01
Singapore 168937
Tel: (65) 6435 3878/9

Child Development Unit

KK Women's and Children's Hospital
Specialist Clinic M Podium I, Children's Tower
100 Bukit Timah Road
Singapore 229899
Tel: (65) 6394 2211

The Children's Specialist Clinic

National University Hospital
Clinic 'A'
Main Building, Level 1
National University Hospital
5 Lower Kent Ridge Road
Singapore 119074
Tel: (65) 6772 5502

Support Groups in Singapore

**The Society for the Promotion of
ADHD Research and Knowledge (SPARK)**
Email: SPARK_Singapore@yahoogroups.com
Website: http://www.spark.org.sg/help.html

Dyslexia Association of Singapore
1 Jurong West Central 2
#05-01 Jurong Point
Singapore 648886
Tel: (65) 6444 5700
Email: info@das.org.sg
Website: www.das.org.sg

Autism Resource Centre (Singapore)
5 Ang Mo Kio Avenue 10
Singapore 569739
Tel: (65) 6323 3258
Email: arc@autism.org.sg
Website: www.autism.org.sg

Autism Association (Singapore)
101 Bukit Batok West Avenue 3
#01-01
Singapore 659168
Tel: (65) 6774 6649
Email: autism@singnet.com.sg
Website: www.autismsg.org

Support Groups in Malaysia

National Autistic Society of Malaysia (NASOM)
NASOM-Kiwanis PJ Autism One-Stop Centre
340 Jalan Pahang
53000 Kuala Lumpur
Tel: (603) 4023 6698
Email: nasomosc@nasom.com.my
Website: www.nasom.com.my

Support Groups in Indonesia

School for Autistic Children
21 Taragong Raya
16 Pondok Indoh
Jakarta

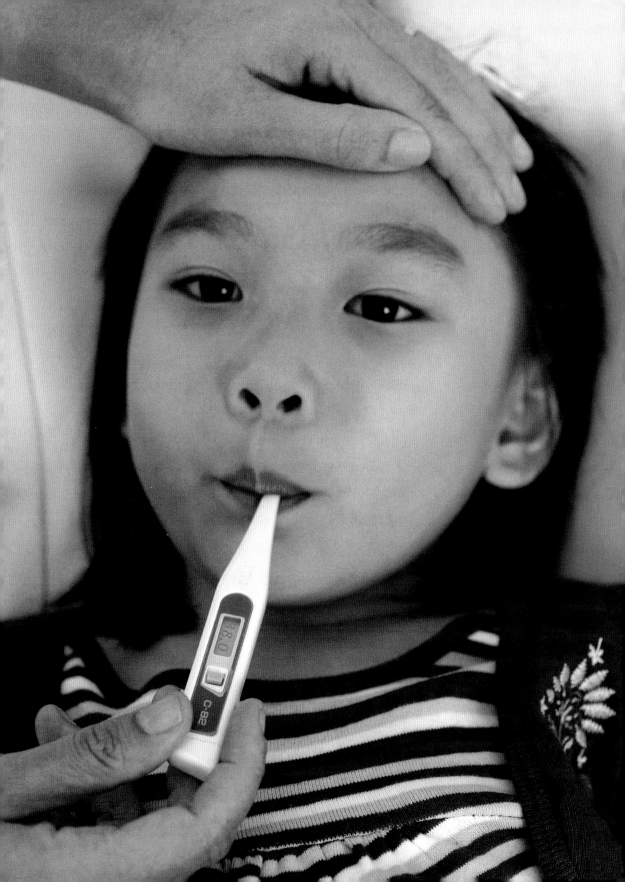

Health Care
and Safety

One of the most important roles of parenting
is to ensure that your child is kept healthy and happy
through his growing years. The health and safety
choices you make for your child will be crucial
in helping him develop physically
and keeping him from serious injury.

Contributors:

Dr Chng Seo Yi
Ms Anna Jacob
Prof Quak Seng Hock
Assoc Prof Lynette Shek
Dr Wendy Sinnathamby
Dr Mas Suhaila Isa

Immunisation

Immunisation (vaccination) protects your child against certain serious infectious diseases. Without immunisation, he is more vulnerable to them. Some vaccines provide prolonged or even lifelong immunity and need to be given just once. Others, however, require repeated injections called boosters in order to maintain the immunity. The programme usually begins at birth.

Childhood Vaccines

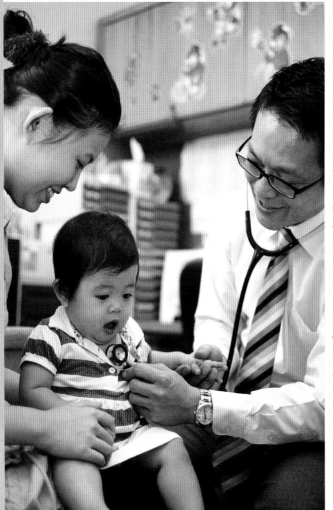

Your child may experience side effects but the risk is low. Consult your doctor if you are concerned about your child's reaction to them. In most children, the side effects of immunisation are mild and go away within a few days. Serious reactions are very rare. The benefits to the child and the community as a whole far outweigh any risks. The important thing to remember is that children are in much more danger from the disease than from the immunisation.

A common side effect of some vaccines is fever, while a few other vaccines may cause rashes. Your doctor will be able to advise you on the side effects of the various vaccines and how to deal with them.

Recommended Childhood Vaccines

The World Health Organization (WHO) recommends a number of standard vaccines to be given to all children. Some of these vaccinations are compulsory either by legislation or by requirement for school enrolment.

Childhood Vaccination Schedule in Singapore

Age	Type of Vaccine	Remarks
Newborns	BCG for tuberculosis (TB) Hepatitis B (1st dose)	Usually given at the hospital with parental consent
1 month	Hepatitis B (2nd dose)	
3 months	Diptheria/Tetanus/Pertussis (DTaP) (1st dose) Poliomyelitis Vaccine (1st dose) Pneumococcal Conjugate Vaccine (1st dose)	Can be given as a combination 5-in-1 vaccine
4 months	Diptheria/Tetanus/Pertussis (DTaP) (2nd dose) Poliomyelitis Vaccine (2nd dose)	
5 months	Diptheria/Tetanus/Pertussis (DTaP) (3rd dose) Poliomyelitis Vaccine (3rd dose) Pneumococcal Conjugate Vaccine (2nd dose)	
5 to 6 months	Hepatitis B (3rd dose)	
12 to 24 months	Measles, Mumps, Rubella (MMR) Pneumococcal Conjugate Vaccine (Booster dose)	Usually given at 15 months
18 months	Diptheria/Pertussis/Tetanus (DTaP) (1st booster) Poliomyelitis Vaccine (1st booster)	
6 to 7 years	Measles, Mumps, Rubella (MMR) Poliomyelitis Vaccine (2nd booster)	
10 to 11 years	Diptheria, Tetanus (DT) (2nd booster) Poliomyelitis Vaccine (3rd booster)	

Vaccines for Potentially Serious Childhood Diseases

BCG Vaccine

In Singapore, newborns in hospitals are given the BCG vaccination routinely as it has been proven to be effective against tuberculosis. Tuberculosis is a disease that not only may cause lung damage but may spread to infect the brain, kidneys and spine. This is the only injection that will leave a scar. You can choose to let your baby have this vaccination on his buttocks or sole of his foot if you do not want him to have a scar on his arm.

Hepatitis B Vaccine

The hepatitis B vaccine protects against the most common cause of chronic liver disease in Singapore. It is given to children at birth, 1 month and 5 to 6 months of age. Boosters may be required after a few years if immunity starts to drop.

DTaP Vaccine

Given as a single injection, DTaP vaccinates against diphtheria, tetanus (lockjaw) and pertussis (whooping cough). These are serious illnesses that can cause death or severe damage to the health of children. The vaccine is given as three doses in the first year of life followed by a booster dose at 18 months.

Side effects of this vaccine include some pain, swelling and redness at the site of the injection. Your child may become a little more fussy or lose his appetite for one or two days. Fever is also fairly common. Some children may have high fevers of more than 39°C. Fever-reducing medicines such as paracetamol will be provided when your child receives this vaccination. More severe reactions are rare.

Polio Vaccine

The polio vaccine (OPV) helps prevent poliomyelitis. This used to be a common cause of paralysis and death. The polio vaccine is given in three doses in the first year of life, followed by booster doses at 18 months, then at around 7 and 11 years of age. It can be given as a live oral vaccine or a killed injectable vaccine.

MMR Vaccine

Vaccination against the following three diseases—measles, mumps, rubella (MMR)—is given as a single injection. These diseases were once very common among children and caused problems ranging from mild symptoms to severe complications like infection of the brain and lungs. This vaccine has an excellent safety record, with fever and rash as the more common side effects. It is given as a single dose at 12 to 24 months and again when your child is 6 years old.

Pneumococcal Vaccine

The pneumococcal vaccine protects children from pneumonia (lung infection), meningitis (brain infection), septicaemia (blood infection) and otitis media (ear infections) caused by the bacteria Streptococcus pneumoniae. It does not protect against all such infections but against the most common and severe causes of bacterial pneumonia and meningitis in Singapore. The pneumococcal vaccine is given in two or three doses in the first year, with a booster between 1 and 2 years of age.

Optional Vaccines

Haemophilus Influenzae Type B (Hib) Vaccine
Serious haemophilus influenzae type B infections can cause meningitis, which can lead to permanent mental and neurological disabilities. It is usually given as part of combined vaccine preparations (5-in-1 or 6-in-1).

Chickenpox Vaccine
Chickenpox is generally considered a mild illness in young children. However, it can be serious and even life threatening in newborns, adults and patients with low immunity. If a child has not had chickenpox by the time he reaches 12 years old, vaccination should be considered as the infection tends to be more severe in adolescents and adults.

Influenza Vaccine
The influenza vaccine protects against flu caused by the influenza virus. This vaccine is particularly popular during the winter season in temperate regions, as epidemics tend to occur at this time. The vaccine has to be given annually as the virus strains change every year. It is recommended for children below 5 years because of their lower immunity.

Rotavirus Vaccine
Rotavirus causes severe fever, diarrhoea and vomiting in young children. The symptoms can last four to eight days and, on occasion, may even persist for up to three weeks. There is no specific treatment for rotaviral infection but your child may be hospitalised if he becomes dehydrated or is unable to retain fluid. The vaccine is given in two or three oral doses, depending on the make, during the first six months of life.

Common Childhood Illnesses

Young babies and children are susceptible to illnesses because their immune systems are not fully developed. A child who is ill may appear pale and listless although most toddlers and preschoolers remain active, going about their tasks as usual. Regardless of how your child reacts to his illness, recognising the symptoms will help you better manage his condition and safeguard his health.

Common Cold

Should your newborn or infant develop a cold, take him to the doctor as it might develop into something more serious like pneumonia. Even without such a complication, a stuffy nose can make it difficult for your baby to nurse or drink from a bottle. This can lead to dehydration, which can be dangerous in babies.

Symptoms of a Common Cold

∗ Congested or runny nose.

∗ Temperature of 38°C or above.

∗ Sneezing.

∗ Coughing.

∗ Decreased appetite or refusal to feed.

∗ Unexplained irritability such as crying and difficulty sleeping.

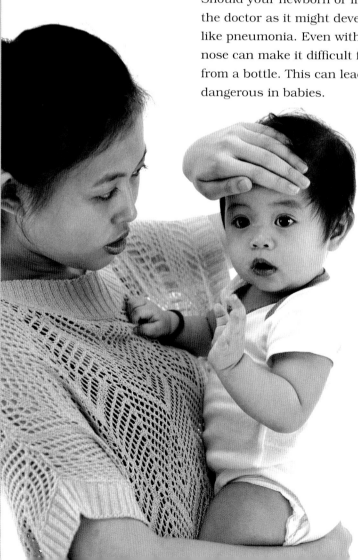

Fever

An unexplained fever may be a cause for concern in infants and young children. Take your child to the doctor if he exhibits any of these symptoms.

Symptoms of Fever

* Temperature of 38°C or above.

* High body temperature and unexplained irritability such as crying.

* Refusal to feed.

* High body temperature, lethargy and unresponsiveness. In infants and children younger than 2 years, these may be signs of meningitis, an infection and inflammation of the membranes and fluid surrounding the brain and spinal cord. If you are worried that your baby may have meningitis, see your doctor immediately.

* Fever lasting for more than a day (for children under 2 years).

* Fever lasting for more than three days (for children 2 years and above).

Febrile Fits

A rapid rise in temperature may cause febrile fits or seizures in some young children under 5 years of age. Although it may be alarming for parents to see their child briefly losing consciousness and convulsing, febrile fits usually cause no harm.

If a seizure occurs, lay your child on his side. Remove any sharp objects near your child, loosen tight clothing and hold your child lightly to prevent injury. Do not place anything in your child's mouth or try to stop the seizure.

Most seizures stop after a few minutes. Call for an ambulance should the seizure last longer than 10 minutes. Take your child to the doctor as soon as possible after the seizure to determine the cause of the fever.

Diarrhoea

Diarrhoea is defined as the passage of three or more loose or liquid stools per day, or more frequently than is normal for your baby. Diarrhoea in babies and young children can be a result of poor hygiene or eating contaminated food. Sometimes, it could be a result of eating new food or a side effect of medication.

Most children lose their appetite when their stomach is upset. Do not force him if he does not want to eat but give him plenty of fluid to drink so he does not become dehydrated. Avoid dairy products like milk and ice cream, as well as fatty, fried and spicy food. See that your child gets enough rest.

Take your child to the doctor immediately if he exhibits any of these symptoms.

Symptoms of Diarrhoea

* Frequent, loose and watery stools.

* Bloody or black stools.

* Fever of 38°C or higher.

Symptoms of Dehydration Caused by Diarrhoea

* Dry mouth and skin, sunken appearance to the abdomen, eyes or cheeks, or crying without tears.

* Not urinated for at least six hours.

* The soft spot (fontanelle) on top of his head is sunken.

* Drowsy, unresponsive or irritable.

Treatment for Diarrhoea

Consult your doctor as soon as possible. Your doctor may recommend an electrolyte solution for rehydration. Do not give your baby antidiarrhoeal medication unless advised by your doctor.

Give your child plenty of fluid, or breastfeed often. If your child is on formula, do not dilute the formula as this will reduce his nutritional intake at a time when his needs are increased. Switch to a product that does not contain lactose such as a soy formula.

Sore Throat (Acute Tonsillitis)

In most cases of the common sore throat, the tonsils, which are situated on both sides near the back of the throat, become infected. It may be caused by a viral or bacterial infection.

Symptoms of Acute Tonsillitis

* Fever.

* Refusal to eat because the tonsils are swollen and painful due to inflammation.

* Runny nose.

* Red eyes.

* Hoarse voice and sore throat.

Treatment for Acute Tonsillitis

If the infection is viral, your doctor will prescribe medication like paracetamol and advise you to give your child a lot of fluid.

If the infection is bacterial, your child is likely to feel quite ill. The doctor may find that his throat is very red and the tonsils may be covered with a whitish coat. In this case, the child will be prescribed antibiotics to shorten the infection period and help prevent complications.

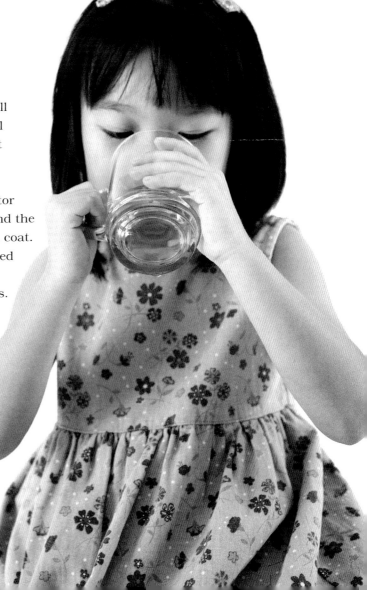

Ear Infection

It is not uncommon for young children to have an ear infection, especially when they catch a cold. This is because the tube in the middle ear that connects the ear to the throat is small and gets blocked easily and germs will grow in the fluid trapped inside.

Symptoms of an Ear Infection

* Pulling at the ears and crying.

* Fever and unexplained irritability.

* Unable to sleep.

Treatment for an Ear Infection

Take your child to the doctor if he exhibits these symptoms. Depending on how bad the infection is, the doctor may prescribe a course of antibiotics as well as a nasal decongestant. The antibiotics will eradicate the bacteria that are causing the infection and the decongestant will unblock the tube in the middle ear.

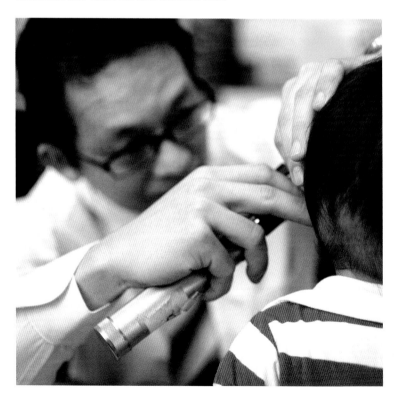

Conjunctivitis (Red Eye)

This is a common and contagious eye infection with seasonal outbreaks. It is an inflammation of the transparent membrane that surrounds the eyeball, causing the eye to be swollen and small blood vessels in the eye to become more prominent, resulting in the 'red' eye.

There are several types of conjunctivitis and they are caused by viruses, bacteria, allergies and chemical irritation. Young children are susceptible to conjunctivitis because of their poor immune defences.

Symptoms of Conjunctivitis

✱ Redness and itchiness in either eye.

✱ A gritty feeling or sandy sensation in either eye.

✱ A whitish/yellowish discharge in either eye that forms a crust during the night.

✱ Watering from either eye.

Treatment for Conjunctivitis

For bacterial conjunctivitis, antibiotic eye drops are used to treat the eye infection and the infection should clear within a few days. Sometimes, an antibiotic eye ointment may be prescribed for treating bacterial red eye in children.

Viral conjunctivitis does not respond to treatment with antibiotic eye drops or ointment. It is self-limiting and may take two to three weeks to clear.

Allergic conjunctivitis is treated with eye drops containing antihistamines, decongestants, mast cell stabilisers, steroids or anti-inflammatory drops. It is best to avoid rubbing the eyes.

Prevention of Conjunctivitis

The best way to control the spread of conjunctivitis caused by infection is by practising good hygiene.

✱ Wash hands thoroughly with soap and water.

✱ Do not touch the eyes.

✱ Change your child's towel, pillowcase and bed sheets often and do not share them with others.

✱ If a child is infected, avoid close contact with other children.

Chickenpox

Chickenpox is a common childhood disease that is highly contagious. There is a vaccine available to protect against the virus, although a small percentage of those who are vaccinated still get chickenpox. In such cases however, the symptoms will be much milder.

How Is Chickenpox Spread?

Chickenpox spreads by direct contact or by droplets from an infected person when he coughs or sneezes. The person is most infectious one or two days before the rash appears until about a week later when the blisters have crusted over and formed scabs. You can get chickenpox within 10 to 21 days after contact with an infected person.

Once you have had chickenpox, you are immune to the disease and are very unlikely to catch it again. However, the virus remains dormant in your nervous system and can cause shingles many years later.

Symptoms of Chickenpox

* An itchy rash resembling insect bites which will turn into blisters that break open and crust over. Common sites for the rash include the face, scalp, chest and back. The rash can also spread across the entire body, and into the throat, eyes and vagina. New spots continue to appear for several days. In healthy children, the disease is generally mild.

* Fever.

* Loss of appetite.

* Mild headache.

* Overall feeling of discomfort and irritability.

Treatment

Treatment for chickenpox is generally to reduce the itch and discomfort. Children with chickenpox should not be given aspirin because of the possibility of causing a complication called Reye's syndrome, a very rare but serious illness that can affect the brain and liver.

There are anti-viral medications that can be used to treat chickenpox. These are usually most effective when taken within the first 24 hours of developing the illness. They reduce the severity and duration of chickenpox and the likelihood of complications.

Prevention

The chickenpox vaccine is safe and effective in protecting those who have never had chickenpox. Although it is not compulsory in Singapore to vaccinate children against chickenpox, it is recommended that you have your child vaccinated when he is between 12 and 18 months.

Children below the age of 13 years receive only a single dose of the chickenpox vaccine. However, those who are 13 years and older need two doses, four to eight weeks apart.

Although chickenpox is a mild disease in children, vaccination is recommended because the symptoms might be more severe should they get it when they are adults. If your child is not vaccinated against chickenpox, he may come down with it during a major examination or other significant event in his life.

Vaccination will also help prevent your child from catching the disease and spreading it to older people or pregnant women for whom the consequences can be devastating.

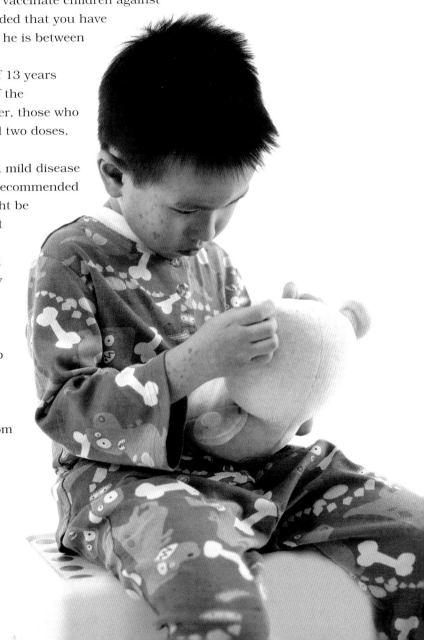

Hand, Foot and Mouth Disease

Hand, foot and mouth disease (HFMD) is a common viral infection. Outbreaks occur most often among preschoolers although older children and adults do get it too. There is no specific treatment for the infection, but children typically recover without treatment after about a week.

Causes of HFMD

HFMD can be caused by a number of viruses, with the most common being the Coxsackie virus and Enterovirus 71. The infection is usually mild but it has been known to cause serious complications and even death, so understand the symptoms and take the necessary precautions.

Symptoms of HFMD

* Mild fever of about 38°C.

* Sore throat.

* Loss of appetite.

* Small, painful ulcers or sores on the tongue, gums and inside of the cheeks.

* Rash that starts out as small red dots and then develops into small blisters on the palms of the hands, soles of the feet and the diaper area.

* Vomiting and/or diarrhoea.

Severe ulcers in the mouth can be painful and this may deter your child from eating and drinking. He may become dehydrated from persistent vomiting/diarrhoea as well as from reduced fluid intake because of the mouth ulcers.

Signs of Complications

Complications such as brain, lung and heart infections may occur occasionally. Signs of complications include:

* Severe headache, giddiness and neck stiffness.

* Disorientation, drowsiness and/or irritability.

* Fits.

* Breathlessness or turning blue.

Treatment of HFMD

If you suspect your child has HFMD, take him to your family doctor who will be able to treat the fever and offer your child some pain relief from the symptoms. You can help ease your child's discomfort by:

* Giving him more fluid.

* Putting him on a soft diet of porridge or pureed fruit if the mouth ulcers are a problem.

* Making sure he takes the medication prescribed by the doctor.

* Keeping him at home.

* Seeing that he gets plenty of rest.

Is it Contagious?

The virus can be transmitted through saliva, fluid from the nose and the blisters as well as stools so it is important that you observe these precautions should your child have HFMD:

* Inform the school, kindergarten or child care centre as soon as possible so they can monitor other children closely and take additional precautions to prevent the spread of HFMD.

* Keep him at home away from school, kindergarten or the child care centre.

* Keep him away from all public places including restaurants, playgrounds and shopping centres.

* Look out for signs and symptoms in other family members, both children and adults.

* Keep his toys, books, eating utensils, towels and clothes separate from others.

* Keep him at home until all the blisters have dried up and he has fully recovered.

Protect Your Child from HFMD

You can protect your child from HFMD by teaching him good personal hygiene.

- Wash his hands properly with soap and water before eating and after going to the toilet.
- Cover his mouth and nose when coughing or sneezing.
- Do not share eating utensils.
- Ensure that toys or appliances that are contaminated by nasal or oral secretions are cleaned thoroughly before they are used again.

Asthma

Asthma is an inflammation of the airways caused by hypersensitivity to a variety of allergens like dust mites, cigarette smoke and animal dander. It causes the airways to narrow, making it difficult to breathe. In Singapore, one in five schoolchildren is asthmatic and it is the main reason for absence from school.

Symptoms of Asthma

Children with asthma may find the symptoms interfering with their sleep and daily activities. These include:

* Coughing.

* A whistling or wheezing sound when exhaling.

* Shortness of breath.

* Chest congestion or tightness.

Triggers for Asthma

The triggers for asthma differ from child to child. Some common triggers include:

* Viral infections such as the common cold.

* Allergens such as dust mites, pet dander, pollen or mould.

* Tobacco smoke or other environmental pollutants.

* Exercise.

* Weather changes or cold air.

Treatment for Asthma

The aim of treatment is to keep the asthma under control. Children whose asthma is well managed can run and play like other children when they are well. If the asthma is not well controlled, it can cause serious if not life-threatening asthma attacks.

The type of treatment prescribed depends on the severity of the child's asthma, symptoms and triggers, and what seems to work best to keep his asthma under control. This includes medication to prevent symptoms and relief medication to quickly open up airways when the child is having an asthma attack. In some cases, medication may be prescribed to treat the allergies.

Prevention of Asthma

The best preventive measures are:

* Avoid triggers. As much as possible, avoid the allergens and irritants that have been identified as triggers for your child's asthma.

* When your child is well, make sure he gets enough exercise. Contrary to what many believe, swimming is good for conditioning the lungs to work more efficiently.

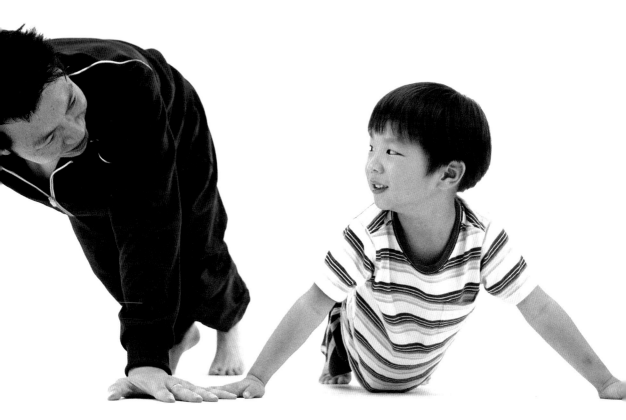

Abdominal Pain

Abdominal pain in children is common and can be distressing to parents, especially when your child is young and unable to describe the pain except by crying. At times, he may double up in pain and break out in a cold sweat.

Abdominal pain in children may be acute or recurrent. Acute abdominal pain comes on suddenly and there may also be other associated symptoms such as nausea, vomiting, fever, distension and diarrhoea. There are many causes of acute abdominal pain, the most common of which is infection.

Bacterial or Viral Infection

The infection may be located in the gastrointestinal or extra-intestinal tract. It is caused by bacteria or a virus entering the body through the mouth. Often, the child will get over the infection within a few days even without medical treatment. Occasionally, antibiotics may be necessary to treat gastrointestinal tract infections that are caused by bacteria.

However, it is important to ensure that your child does not become dehydrated. Continue to feed him normally and check his urine output. Most healthy children urinate at least two or three times in the morning and another two or three times in the afternoon. A decrease in urine output means that your child is dehydrated and you should take him to the doctor.

If your child is still drinking from the bottle, make sure that the bottle and the rubber teat are cleaned properly. Inculcate in your child, from young, the importance of personal hygiene such as hand-washing after visiting the toilet and before touching food.

Acute Appendicitis

The signs of acute appendicitis are abdominal pain and fever, and sometimes also painful urination. At first, the pain is centred around the belly button. As the appendicitis progresses, the pain shifts to the right side of the lower abdomen. If not operated in time, the appendix can become gangrenous and perforate. By this stage, the patient can become very sick and it may be fatal.

Intussusception

Intussusception is a condition when a segment of the intestine slides into another segment, like a telescope. The abdominal pain is similar to that of colic, followed by vomiting and distension of the stomach. As it gets worse, the child may pass bloody jelly-like stools. By this time, it is an emergency situation and you should take your child to the hospital immediately to correct the 'telescoping' intestine, or the affected portion of the intestine may become infected.

Urinary Tract Infection

This is another common cause of acute abdominal pain in children. The signs are pain in the lower abdomen and during urination, and sometimes also fever. Often, antibiotics are necessary to treat the urinary tract infection (UTI) and imaging of the tract may be done to check for abnormalities in the kidneys or bladder. Untreated, a UTI can lead to acute or chronic kidney infection, which can permanently damage the kidneys.

Constipation

This is a common cause of recurrent abdominal pain. The symptoms are infrequent bowel movements or passage of dry, hard stools. Make sure that your child has enough fibre in his diet by giving him more fruit and vegetables, and encourage him to consume more fluid. Although this is usually not serious, take your child to the doctor if the constipation lasts longer than two weeks.

Lactose Intolerance

Lactose intolerance is common in Asian children. The abdominal pain comes on a few hours after consuming food containing lactose. The abdomen may also feel distended and there is increase in flatulence. Stop giving your child dairy products or substitute with low lactose dairy products or soy milk and the pain will go away.

Peptic Ulcers

Occasionally, children may suffer from gastric diseases such as peptic ulcers, which is an infection of the stomach by bacteria called Helicobacter pylori. The pain is located in the upper abdomen and is aggravated by food or hunger. Medical attention should be sought so that the infection can be treated with appropriate medication.

Gastroesophageal Reflux

This is another common cause of recurrent abdominal pain. The location of pain is similar to that of peptic ulcer disease, in the upper abdomen. The pain is worse after eating a full meal. This is due to laxity of the valve at the lower end of the food pipe, resulting in the back flow of stomach acid. The stomach acid causes injuries to the lower end of the food pipe, hence the pain. Occasionally, this may be due to other more serious abnormalities of the lower end of the food pipe and surgery may be necessary. In children with gastroesophageal reflux, small, frequent feeds often help to improve the symptoms. A course of acid-reducing medicine would be needed in severe cases.

Chronic Inflammatory Bowel Disease

This inflammation of the gastrointestinal tract used to be more common among the Caucasian community, but it is now becoming more common in Singapore. A prominent symptom is abdominal pain. There may be other symptoms like loss of appetite, loss of weight and diarrhoea with blood in the stools. Endoscopy and imaging of the gastrointestinal tract are necessary for proper diagnosis. The treatment is long term.

Chronic Constipation

The most common cause of constipation in children is a lack of fluid and fibre in the diet. The child's stools become hard and he experiences pain or discomfort when passing the hard stool. The pain is worsened when there is blood in the stool as this means there has been a tear within the anal canal caused by the hard stool.

In time, the child with on-going constipation will associate passing motion with pain and start to withhold moving his bowels. What parents usually interpret as the child straining when passing motion is, in fact, the child trying to stop the stool from coming out.

Some children may refuse to sit on the toilet bowl or potty and may take on abnormal postures to do this. With worsening constipation, the rectum (the part of the intestine where stool is stored) increasingly distends and eventually the child will lose the urge to pass motion, making his constipation go from bad to worse.

Managing Your Child's Constipation

Diet

* Ensure that your child has a daily diet rich in wholegrains, fruit and vegetables.

* Encourage your child to drink more water.

Bowel Training

* Encourage your child to go to the toilet when he feels the urge to pass motion. You will be able to recognise the urge by his behaviour.

* Encourage him to sit on the toilet seat for at least 10 minutes every day at the same time, preferably after a meal. Ideally, get your child to sit on the toilet with his legs resting on a stool to provide more stability and comfort. Get him to relax by reading a book.

Laxatives

✳ Laxatives play an important role in treating children with chronic constipation. The aim of using laxatives is to bulk up the stool and make it soft, thus ensuring that passing motion is as painless as possible. Children who have lost the urge to pass motion will need a stimulant laxative. Do not give your child laxatives on your own. The use of laxatives should be guided by your doctor. Some children might need to be on laxatives for six months to two years.

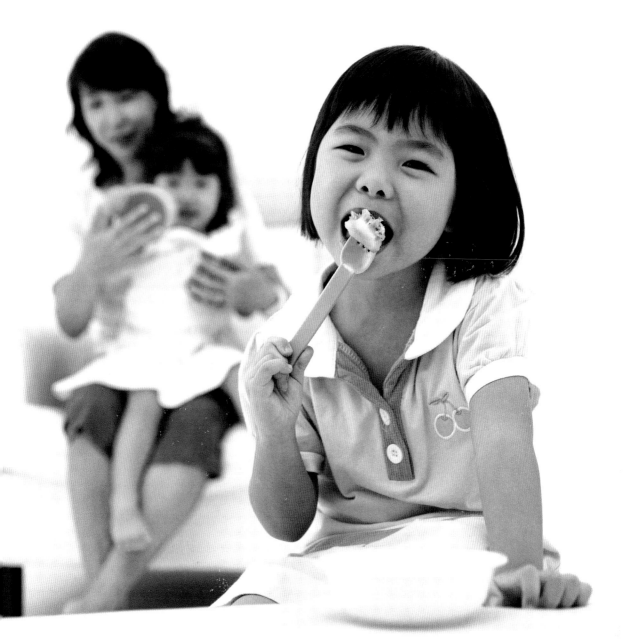

Food Allergies

Food allergies affect 4 to 5 percent of children in Singapore. Sometimes, it is hard to distinguish between a true food allergy and a food intolerance. By definition, an allergy involves the immune system while an intolerance (such as lactose intolerance) does not.

Symptoms of allergies can be mild but, at times, they can cause rashes, digestive and respiratory conditions and, on the rare occasion, even death. Prevention, accurate diagnosis and treatment are important to prevent children from suffering unnecessarily. Take care not to impose unnecessary diet restrictions on your child if he has a food allergy as this is very hard to adhere to and may also cause nutritional deficiencies in the long term.

Eggs, milk, peanuts, wheat, soy and certain types of seafood, including prawns and fish, are common causes of food allergies in children. This is because their bodies react adversely to the proteins in the food.

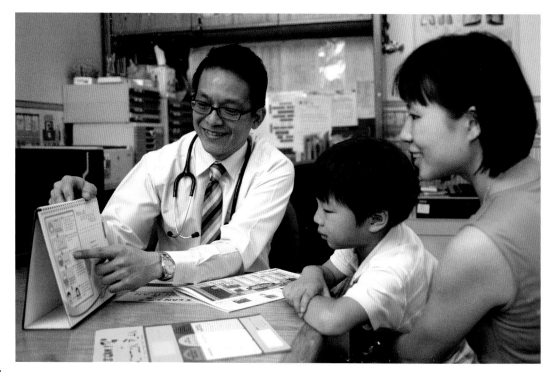

The symptoms of a food allergy include:

* Tingling in the mouth.

* Hives, itching or eczema.

* Swelling of the lips, face, tongue and throat, or other parts of the body.

* Wheezing, nasal congestion or trouble breathing.

* Abdominal pain, diarrhoea, nausea or vomiting.

* Dizziness, light-headedness or fainting.

* In severe cases, a food allergy can cause anaphylactic shock, a very sudden and serious allergic reaction. The symptoms can be fatal without immediate medical treatment.

Prevention

A food allergy is more likely to occur in your child if you have a family history of atopic disease (eczema, asthma and rhinoconjunctivitis). Prevention is better than cure. At this time, the best practices supported by science are:

Exclusive Breastfeeding
If your child is at high risk of developing an allergy, providing him with only breast milk alone for four to six months may be beneficial.

Extensively Hydrolysed or Partially Hydrolysed Formulas
If breastfeeding is not possible, hydrolysed formulas where the proteins are partially broken down for easier digestion, such as extensively hydrolysed casein or partially hydrolysed whey, may help in the prevention of atopy.

Delayed Introduction of Complementary Food
Solid food should be introduced to the diet only after the child is 6 months old. Introduce potential allergens only when your child is older, such as cow's milk at 12 months, eggs at 2 years and nuts and fish at 3 years.

Treatment

There is no better treatment for a food allergy than complete avoidance of the trigger.

Cow's Milk Protein Allergy

If your child is taking a cow's milk-based formula, your doctor might suggest replacing it with a soy-based formula. If your child is still not able to tolerate that, he might suggest an extensively hydrolysed formula (eHF) or amino acid-based formula. The effects should be seen within two to four weeks. Continue with the formula until the cow's milk allergy is overcome.

Note: Partially hydrolysed formula is not suitable for infants with cow's milk allergy. Goat's or sheep's milk are also not suitable for infants with cow's milk allergy.

Lactose Intolerance

Lactose or milk sugar is found in milk and milk products such as yoghurt and cheese. All forms of mammalian milk—human, cow, sheep and goat—contain lactose. Lactose is a double sugar, made up of glucose and galactose. An enzyme, lactase, in our small intestine splits lactose into the individual sugars before they are absorbed.

Lactose intolerance is very common in Asians. In those who are lactose intolerant, the small intestine does not produce lactase or does not produce sufficient lactase. This results in lactose passing undigested through the gut to the large intestine.

Symptoms

Lactose intolerance is accompanied by abdominal pain, diarrhoea, nausea, flatulence and/or bloating after the ingestion of lactose or lactose-containing food substances. Sometimes, infants develop secondary lactase deficiency as a result of small bowel injury, such as acute gastroenteritis, persistent diarrhoea or other causes of injury to the small intestinal wall. This can happen at any age but is more common in infancy.

Treatment

Avoid dairy products that contain lactose such as milk, yoghurt and cheese to alleviate the symptoms. However, discontinued consumption of such products may cause deficiency of calcium, vitamin D and other nutrients over time. Offer your child a soy formula that is naturally lactose-free or a low lactose formula. To help your child achieve his calcium needs, offer him other food rich in calcium such as soy bean curd, green leafy vegetables and lentils.

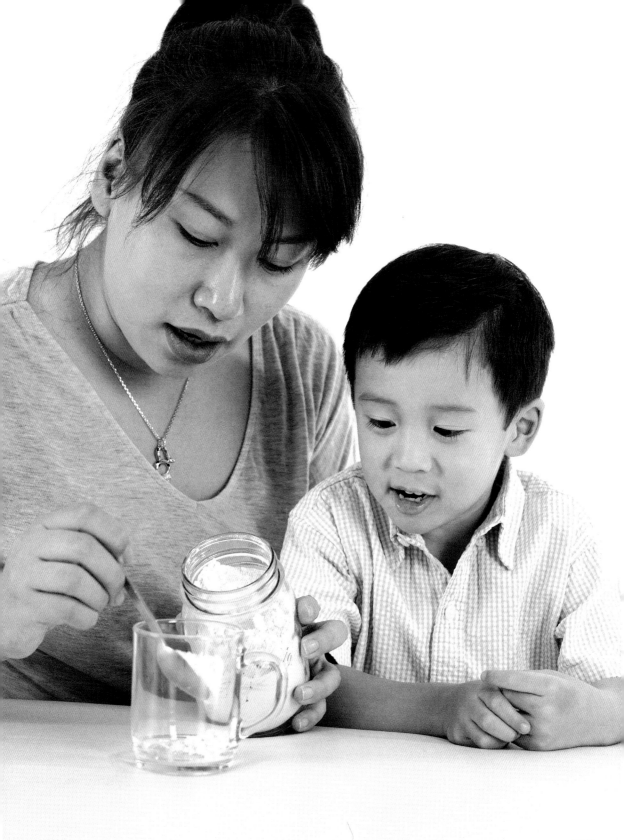

Sleep

Good sleep is as important as good nutrition for the physical and mental development of your young child. Young children need to have sufficient sleep and good quality sleep. Sleep is important for the development of the immune system, heart and blood vessels and hormonal function in children. Just as you actively plan for enrichment classes for your child, do not forget to set aside time for him to play and rest.

Importance of Naps for Young Children

Contrary to popular belief, skipping or withholding naps in a younger child will not facilitate sleep at bedtime but can be counterproductive and result in the child becoming overtired and having more difficulty falling asleep and staying asleep.

Develop Healthy Sleep Habits

Help your child develop a consistent and age-appropriate sleep-wake schedule. His bedtime and wake time should be at about the same time every day. There should be no more than a one- to two- hour difference between weekday and weekend bedtimes and wake times.

An age-appropriate bedtime is an essential component of this schedule. Earlier bedtimes are appropriate for your young child in response to his need for more sleep. If your young child's bedtime is too late, he will become overtired, resulting in hyperactivity and irritability.

Regular scheduled naps are important for your young child but avoid very long naps, too many naps or naps in the evening. Naps should be geared to your child's age and developmental needs.

It is important that everyone in the family understands the importance of your child's sleep schedule and adheres to it.

Amount of Sleep a Child Needs

Age	Average Sleep Duration in a 24-hour Period	Sleep Patterns
Newborns	16 to 20 hours in total	1- to 4-hour sleep periods followed by 1- to 2-hour awake periods Amount of daytime sleep equals the amount of night-time sleep
0 to 12 months	13 to 15 hours in total	Day/night differentiation develops between 6 weeks and 3 months Sleeps through the night at 9 months Naps 2 to 4 hours in 2 naps per day
12 months to 3 years	12 hours in total	Naps 1½ to 3½ hours in a single nap per day
3 to 6 years	11 to 12 hours in total	Napping declines Most stop taking naps by 5 years

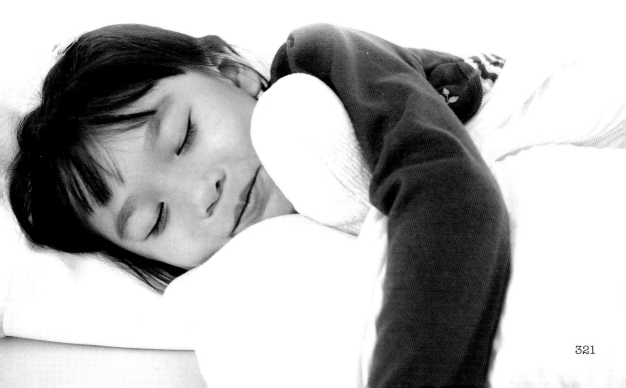

BEDTIME ROUTINE

Your young child should have a consistent bedtime routine of about 30 minutes that consists of the same three to four relaxing activities every night, with the last part of the routine taking place in the room where your child sleeps.

Here is an example of an age-appropriate sleep-wake schedule and bedtime routine for a 10-month-old baby.

7:30 am	Wakes up happy and ready to feed
7:45 am	Breakfast
8:00 am	Plays outside
10:00 am	Milk feed
10:45 am	Morning nap
12:15 pm	Wakes up happy
12:30 pm	Lunch
1:15 pm	Bath
1:30 pm	Plays inside
3:00 pm	Milk feed
3:30 pm	Afternoon nap
5:00 pm	Wakes up happy
5:30 pm	Dinner
6:00 pm	Plays
7:00 pm	Begins bedtime routine
	Bath and change into pyjamas
	Milk feed
	Reading by parents in bedroom
7:45 pm	Lights off and sleeps independently

Sleeping Tips

Start winding down an hour before bedtime. Cease high-energy activities like playing hide-and-seek or running around before bedtime. Also, avoid stimulating activities like watching TV and playing computer games. Spend some quality time every night with your child before putting him to bed, talking and sharing about your day. This will also help you build a bond with your child. Do not use the TV or computer as your child's companion before bedtime. Other tips for better sleep:

Bedroom
Keep your child's bedroom comfortable, quiet, cool and dark. Avoid using your child's bedroom for time out or other punishments.

Bed
Use the bed only for sleeping. Avoid snacking, reading, watching TV or playing on the bed.

TV
Do not have a TV set in your child's bedroom.

Exercise
Get your child to spend some time playing outdoors, especially in the mornings. He will not only be able to expend some energy but will also gain exposure to sunlight to help his body produce vitamin D, an essential vitamin in developing strong bones.

Caffeine
Avoid giving your child food or drink containing caffeine (such as chocolates and cola) at least three to four hours before bedtime.

Snacks
Do not eat too close to bedtime. Any heavy meal should be eaten at least two hours beforehand. If your child is hungry, give him a light snack such as a drink of warm milk.

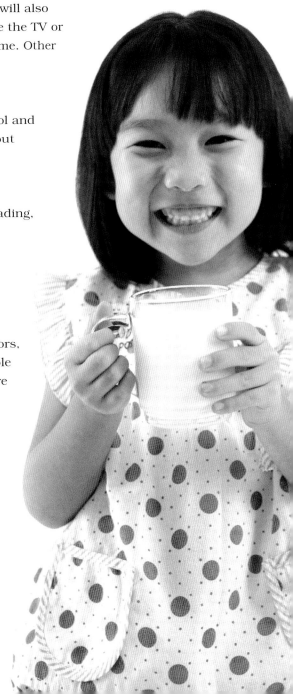

Sleep Disorders

Sleep problems are common in babies and young children. In Singapore, snoring occurs in more than 25 percent of children and obstructive sleep apnoea (OSA) occurs in 1 to 3 percent of children.

Impact on Mental Development

Sleep problems can affect mental development as well as learning in babies and young children. Snoring in babies is associated with decreased scores on the mental development index (MDI) when such snoring induces awakenings and causes disruption in sleep (sleep fragmentation). Living in a smoking household with secondhand exposure to cigarette smoke may also increase the harmful effects of infant snoring.

It has been found that children with lower academic performance in secondary school were more likely to have had snoring problems during early childhood that required treatment. These findings support the concept that the learning deficit may be only partially reversible and that a learning debt may develop with sleep disordered breathing during early childhood and hamper school performance in later years.

Impact on Behaviour

Sleep disorders can cause behavioural problems in children and the reverse is also true. Up to a third of all children with frequent loud snoring or sleep disordered breathing display significant hyperactivity and inattention. It is recommended that children with mild symptoms of ADHD be screened for snoring and other symptoms of OSA as those who have undergone treatment for sleep disordered breathing showed significant improvement in hyperactive and inattentive behaviour.

Common Sleep Problems

Babies and young children can and should be trained to fall asleep on their own without breastfeeding, sucking on a bottle or having their parents sing to them, pat or rock them.

Sleep Onset Association Disorder

Babies who have sleep onset association disorder are unable to fall asleep on their own at bedtime or self-soothe themselves back to sleep during night awakenings without parental intervention. They will wake and cry several times during the night and need the same associations—the breast, bottle or rocking to fall back to sleep. These multiple awakenings affect the sleep quality of both the parent and child and can be a source of emotional stress especially for first-time parents.

Dealing with Sleep Onset Association Disorder

Behavioural treatment is effective in sleep onset association disorder. The two most common approaches used are the standard extinction approach and the graduated extinction approach.

* Standard extinction approach. The baby is allowed to cry to sleep independently in the cot. The time for the baby to cry to sleep can seem an eternity to many parents, so parents who choose this approach must be firm in their conviction.

* Graduated extinction approach. The parents check on their child at fixed intervals, starting with every 5 minutes and progressively increase the interval, until the child falls back to sleep.

The goal of both approaches is to enable the baby or child to develop self-soothing skills so that he can fall asleep independently without negative sleep associations. Both approaches typically take three to seven nights, with the graduated extinction approach taking longer. Once a child learns to fall asleep independently at bedtime, he will also be able to fall asleep independently when he wakes up in the middle of the night.

Limit Setting Sleep Disorder

Limit setting sleep disorder typically occurs in toddlers who are able to walk, run and speak well. These children test the patience of their parents by refusing or delaying their bedtimes. They will try all kinds of delay tactics such as

> **Children with Special Needs**
>
> Sleep problems such as night wakings, early morning wakings and shorter total sleep time are common in children with special needs, in particular children with ADHD, autism spectrum disorders and mood/anxiety disorders.

"Can you read me another story please?", "I'm thirsty. I need a drink" and "I need to go to the toilet." They cry and throw a tantrum if you refuse to accede to their requests.

Dealing with Limit Setting Sleep Disorder
In limit setting sleep disorder, it is important for the parents to be firm and consistent about the bedtime routine and bedtime. Giving in will reinforce the child's delay tactics. Parents need to demonstrate their authority and set the proper limits.

Night Terrors and Nightmares
Night terrors occur early in the sleep period from one to four hours after falling asleep. Children with night terrors can appear very distressed, waking with their eyes wide open while screaming. These children may be sweating, breathing fast and have a rapid heartbeat. During a night terror, the child will appear confused, be unable to recognise the caregiver and be inconsolable. Children with night terrors are unable to recall the event the following morning.

Night terrors are often triggered in young children who are overtired, emotionally stressed or physically unwell. Treatment involves adequate rest and good sleep practices. For frequent night terrors, waking the child before the usual time that he has a night terror may help to prevent it from happening.

Nightmares are frightening dreams triggered by unpleasant experiences. They can be prevented by decreasing stimulating activities at bedtime including watching scary TV programmes. Usually, nightmares occur later in the sleep period at around dawn. Children with nightmares are able to recognise their caregiver and be comforted by their presence. They may be able to relate the frightening dream the following morning.

Obstructive Sleep Apnoea
Snoring is a symptom of airway obstruction during sleep and it can be a manifestation of a more sinister sleep problem known as obstructive sleep apnoea (OSA). In OSA, there is abnormal breathing during sleep with complete or partial airway obstruction that disrupts normal oxygen and carbon dioxide exchange during sleep, leading to disrupted sleep patterns.

Parents of children who habitually snore should consult a paediatrician specialising in sleep disorders. These children may require an overnight sleep study to assess if they have OSA. Children who have OSA should receive treatment as soon as possible. Treatment is usually surgical removal of the tonsils and adenoidal tissues. Preschoolers with OSA show normalised sleep and respiratory patterns and improved cognitive scores following treatment.

Untreated OSA in children can result in high blood pressure and heart strain. OSA can also affect mental development in babies and learning and school performance in children. OSA may also be the cause of mild ADHD symptoms. Thus, children with mild ADHD should be screened for symptoms of OSA.

Preventing Sleep Disorders

Many sleep disorders are preventable if parents take pains to develop good sleeping habits in their young children.

Fortunately, most sleep disorders in children are treatable. These may include medication for narcolepsy (excessive sleepiness in the day), surgery for OSA and behaviour therapy for night-wakings. Often, treatment of the underlying sleep disorder can reverse any related emotional, behavioural or learning disorder in young children.

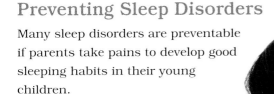

DOES MY CHILD HAVE A SLEEP DISORDER?

Screen your children for sleep disorders with BEARS.

B   **Bedtime Issues.** Does your child have any problem going to bed or any problem falling asleep?

E   **Excessive Daytime Sleepiness.** Does your child show any symptom of excessive daytime sleepiness (sleepy in day and/or difficulty waking up in the morning)? It is important to understand that daytime sleepiness manifests differently at various ages. A baby will be sleepy and tired, a young child will be cranky, irritable and hyperactive and an older child will be lethargic.

A   **Awakenings.** Does your child awaken during the night or have unusual behaviour during the night?

R   **Regularity and Duration of Sleep.** Does your child have a regular sleep schedule and does he get enough sleep?

S   **Snoring.** Does your child snore or have any problem breathing during the night?

Adapted from *A Clinical Guide to Paediatric Sleep* by Jodi A Mindell and Judith A Owens, page 209

Any abnormality on the BEARS screening should prompt the parents to take their baby or child for evaluation by a paediatrician. The paediatrician can then ask more questions, perform a physical examination and, if necessary, request for a sleep diary or an overnight sleep study.

TEETH GRINDING

Teeth grinding or bruxism is common in children. As many as 10 to 20 percent of children below the age of 10 years may grind their teeth during sleep. However, most of them will outgrow this condition before adulthood.

Bruxism usually does not disrupt the sleep of the child. In most cases, treatment is not needed.

However, if the teeth grinding is severe and associated with teeth pain, jaw ache, headaches or wearing out of the teeth, the following measures may be useful:

☐ Get your child to sleep on his side.

☐ Reduce your child's daytime stress or anxiety as this has been found to aggravate bruxism.

☐ Establish a relaxing bedtime routine for your child prior to sleep.

☐ Take your child for a dental evaluation to detect and correct jaw problems or dental malocclusion.

☐ If necessary, your dentist may advise you to get a mouth guard or dental splint made for your child to wear when he sleeps to prevent dental erosion.

☐ Take your child for a sleep evaluation by a paediatric sleep specialist, as bruxism is known to be more common in the presence of other sleep problems like sleep apnoea or nocturnal myoclonus, where a person moves his limbs involuntarily while asleep.

Eye Care

A study conducted by the Singapore National Eye Centre found that the prevalence of myopia in Singapore is the highest in the world. Findings from another study highlight that about 30 percent of children in Singapore have myopia by the time they are 7 years old.

Causes of Myopia

The causes of myopia are not known but studies have found that children with a parent with myopia are more likely to have myopia themselves, especially if they do not practise good eye care habits.

Good Eye Care Habits

Studies have shown that spending some time on outdoor activities every day may help to prevent the development and progression of myopia. Instil in your young child good eye care habits from young.

* Remind your child to take a break from reading, writing and watching TV every 30 minutes by looking at something in the distance.

* Discourage your child from playing for long hours with mobile phone or computer games and provide opportunities for him to play outdoor instead.

Wearing Spectacles

Parents and grandparents often have negative feelings about young children wearing spectacles. It would be wise to keep these feelings to yourselves.

A child will happily accept that he has to wear spectacles if he is introduced to them positively. If your child has to wear spectacles, let him have some say in the choice of the frames.

He will naturally be conscious of the glasses when he first starts wearing them, so a good suggestion is to plan activities to keep him busy for a few days to take his mind off them until he gets used to them.

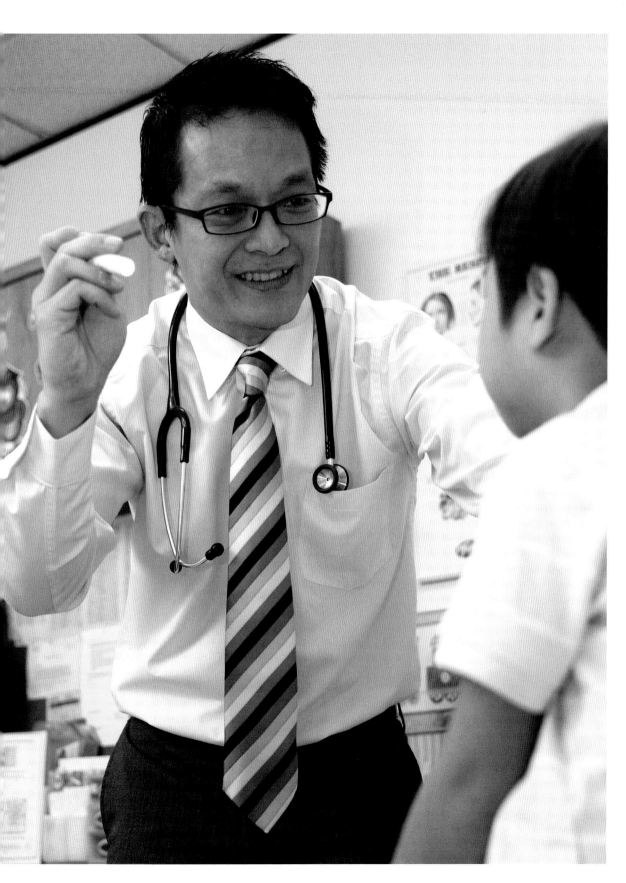

Safety

Statistics show that most childhood injuries are due to accidents in the home. Being aware of the dangers and childproofing your home will help you to prevent these accidents from occurring and reduce the risk of injury at home.

Baby Walker

This wheeled device allows babies to propel themselves with their feet, even before they can walk, and has been responsible for many home accidents.

If you want to get a baby walker for your baby, be sure to keep him away from staircases, stoves and electrical gadgets or anything else that he can reach out for and hurt himself with.

Safety at Home

Children are curious by nature. Young babies and toddlers will touch and tug at anything that catches their eye, and if it looks tempting enough, they will put it into their mouths. Look around your home for hidden dangers and keep them away from your child.

Bedroom

* When purchasing a cot, ensure that the space between the cot slats are 6 cm or less to prevent your baby's head or limbs from getting wedged in between, which could result in strangulation or injury.

* Check that the cot slats are sturdy. Ensure that there are no sharp or protruding edges.

* Check that the locks and latches on the drop-side of the cot have a safety feature such as a double release mechanism so your baby cannot accidentally release the catch and fall out.

* The mattress should fit snugly into the cot so there is no danger of your baby getting caught and wedged in between the mattress and cot, which could result in suffocation.

* Choose a high-density foam mattress, not a spring mattress which has inner parts that can break and injure your baby. Spring mattresses are also thicker and your baby can climb out of the cot more easily once he is more mobile.

* Some modern versions of the sarong cradle come with a motorised spring that will rock your baby to sleep. Babies seem to take to the snug cradling of the sarong cradle but health and baby care experts do not recommend its use as it puts your baby at risk of head injuries if he falls out of it.

Bathroom

* Use a baby bathtub with a non-slip surface or put a non-slip bath mat in the tub to prevent your baby from slipping into the water.

* Test the temperature of the bath water before putting your baby in. Do this by dipping your elbow into the water. It should be comfortably warm and not too hot. Keep the water level shallow.

* Do not let your child play with the shower hose or taps as he may accidentally turn on the hot water and scald himself.

* Never leave your baby unattended in the bathtub, not even for a few seconds to answer the phone or doorbell.

* Never leave buckets or basins with water in them as your child could fall in and drown.

* If you are using cloth diapers and safety pins, open the safety pins and poke the sharp ends into the mattress before changing your baby. You can then easily reach for the pins and your baby will not be in danger of being pricked by the sharp pins.

Kitchen

* Keep your child out of the kitchen, especially when you are cooking.

* Turn in pot handles on the stove to prevent your child from reaching out and pulling them down.

Around the House

* Keep medicines and poisonous substances such as rat poison, aerosols, bleach, washing detergent and other chemicals out of reach.

* Make sure that the cords of electrical appliances are out of reach.

* Place safety covers over all unused power points if they are low enough for your child to poke his fingers into.

* Screen and bar all windows and make sure that the grilles are kept locked.

Jealous Siblings

The arrival of a new baby can evoke feelings of jealousy in your older children, especially those 3 years and under.

Just as a precaution, never leave your baby alone with the older child as he may take it out on the baby, hurting him. Let your older child play and touch his sibling only in your presence.

* Keep all sharp objects like scissors and knives out of reach.

* Make sure that your furniture does not have sharp edges. Ensure all pieces of furniture are solid and heavy, and will not easily tip over should your baby pull on any of them.

* Keep plastic bags away from your child to prevent suffocation.

* Immediately wipe up spilt liquids which may cause your child to slip and fall.

* Keep anything breakable out of your child's reach to avoid him cutting himself on the sharp edges.

* If you have house plants, make sure they are not poisonous.

Safety at Play

Children can get very engrossed in playing which may lead them to getting cuts and bruises from falling or tripping over toys, or when they are not properly supervised while playing outdoors. Be aware of the potential hazards and keep them at bay.

Toys

Although most toys are made with safety in mind, no toy is totally safe. Toys that break or are misused can be dangerous. Likewise, toys that may be safe for older children may be a hazard for younger ones. Always read the safety label on toys and follow the instructions provided. Here are some toy safety tips:

* Age-appropriate toys. Buy toys that are appropriate for your child's age and stage of development.

* Choking hazard. Toys with small parts are not suitable for children under 3 years of age. When buying stuffed toys, check that the small parts such as the eyes, ears and nose will not come off easily. Never give your young child a balloon and leave him unsupervised as the balloon can block his airway if he puts it into his mouth.

* Strangulation hazard. Remove any cot mobiles when your child is old enough to push himself up and reach out for it. Avoid buying toys with cords that are more than 30 cm long to prevent accidental strangulation.

* Sharp points and edges. Avoid toys with sharp points and edges as these can cause serious injuries.

* Battery-operated toys. Make sure that the battery compartment cannot be easily pried open. Small batteries such as mercury disc batteries can be dangerous if your child chokes or swallows them or stuffs them in his ears or up his nose. Remove the batteries in toys when not in use. Batteries that are left in the toys for extended periods of time will leak, and this liquid is poisonous.

* Shooting toys. It is best to avoid these toys because they can cause injury, especially to the eyes.

Water Safety

Make sure that your child is supervised by a responsible adult at all times when swimming. Children have been known to drown when the attention of the adult with them is diverted, even for a short while.

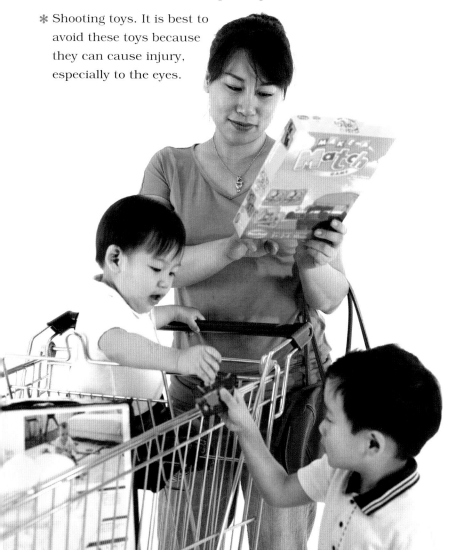

* Noisy toys. Do not choose toys that are very noisy as they may damage your child's hearing.

* Painted toys. Avoid such toys as the paint may come off if your child puts the toy into his mouth.

* Electronic toys. If necessary, get the salesperson to do a demonstration before you decide whether it is safe to purchase the toy.

* Check toys. Go through your child's toy basket regularly to check for breakages. Discard broken toys.

* Store toys properly. Make sure that toys are put away after playing to prevent anyone from stepping on or tripping over them.

Garden

* If you have a garden, pull out any poisonous weeds or fungi whenever they appear.

* Never leave a paddling pool with water in it as your child could fall in and drown.

* Keep garden tools and fertilisers out of your child's reach.

* Make sure the garden gate is always secured so your child cannot wander from the garden onto the road.

* Cover up drains to prevent your child from falling in.

Bicycles

* When getting a bicycle for your child, ensure that it is the right fit for his weight, height and age. Adjust the seat so that his knees are slightly bent when the pedal is at its lowest point.

* Check the bicycle regularly to ensure that the tyres are properly inflated, the brakes work, the chain is tight and lubricated, and the reflectors are in place.

* Have him wear a helment that fits snugly. If you can slip in two fingers on each side of your child's temple, then it is too big for him.

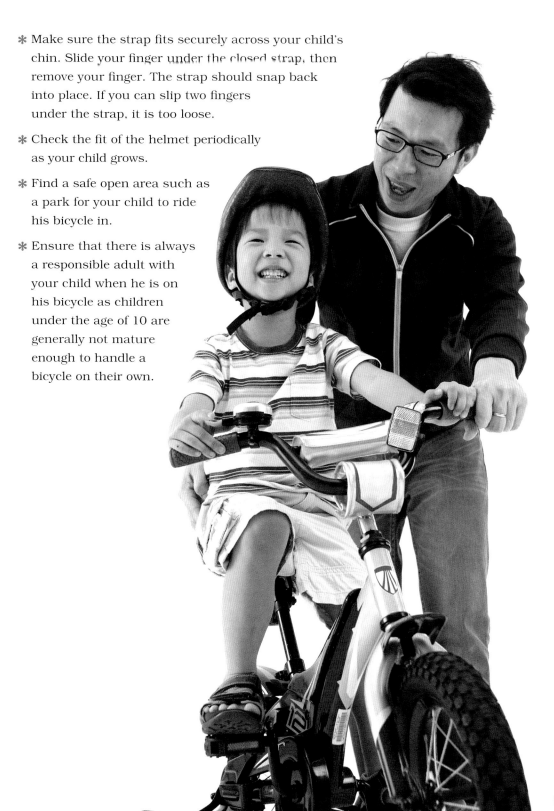

* Make sure the strap fits securely across your child's chin. Slide your finger under the closed strap, then remove your finger. The strap should snap back into place. If you can slip two fingers under the strap, it is too loose.

* Check the fit of the helmet periodically as your child grows.

* Find a safe open area such as a park for your child to ride his bicycle in.

* Ensure that there is always a responsible adult with your child when he is on his bicycle as children under the age of 10 are generally not mature enough to handle a bicycle on their own.

Car Safety

Always ensure that your child is safely strapped into his child seat when travelling in a car. Ensure that the child safety lock is applied so your child will not be able to unlock and open the car door by himself at any time. Never allow your child to stick his head, hands or arms out of the window, and check that his limbs and fingers are safely inside the car before closing the door.

Age	Weight	Type of Restraint
Up to 9 months	Up to 10 kg	Infant capsule
9 months to 4 years	9 to 18 kg	Convertible or forward-facing seat
5 to 8 years	19 to 36 kg	Booster seat

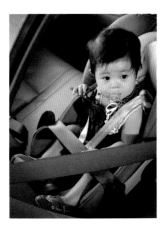

Infant Capsules

The recommended car seat for babies up to 10 kg is a rear-facing infant seat as they offer greater protection for your baby's head, neck and spine.

Infant car seats come with many different features, from detachable bases to five-point harnesses and overhead shields that can be fitted with a canopy to provide additional sun shade. Some features are for additional comfort and some for convenience of use. Scout around for an infant capsule that suits your needs.

Convertible Seats

Convertible seats are suitable for larger infants who may not be able to fit comfortably into infant capsules. Convertible seats can be fitted to be rear-facing as well as forward-facing. Once your child reaches the appropriate weight and size, the convertible seat should be turned around to be forward-facing. Like infant capsules, most convertible seats have a five-point harness.

Forward-facing Seats

Most forward-facing seats come with a five-point harness that will secure your child firmly in his seat and prevent him from sliding under or out of the harness, should there be a crash.

Forward-facing seats can be fitted in the front or rear passenger seats, but it is safer to put them in the rear, especially if there is a passenger airbag in the front.

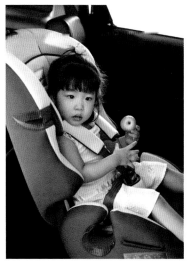

Booster Seat

Booster seats help raise your child's height to a suitable level, enabling him to use adult seat belts safely.

You may want to check out booster seats that come with a back as these will provide your child who has just outgrown his forward-facing seat with a better fit for the seat belt. Always ensure that your child is safely secured in his booster seat.

✳ Fasten the seat belt as tightly as possible.

✳ The lap belt should go over the hips, not the stomach.

✳ The diagonal strap should rest over the shoulder.

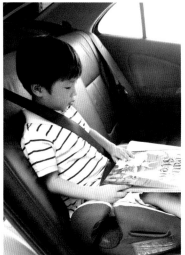

Index

Resources

BOOKS

General Reading for Preschoolers

ABC books

A Mother Goose book of nursery rhymes

Counting books

Dr Seuss books

The Berenstain Bears series by Stan and Jan Berenstain

How do I…? books by Shigeo Watanabe

The *Spot* series by Eric Hill

Books by Eric Carle, such as *The Very Hungry Caterpillar*

Are You My Mother? by P D Eastman

Can't You Sleep Little Bear? by Martin Waddell

Caps for Sale by Esphyr Slobodkina

Dear Zoo by Rod Campbell

Each Peach Pear Plum by Janet and Allen Ahlberg

Little Red Hen

Owl Babies by Martin Waddell

Rhyming Round Bangkok by Kathleen Chia and Linda Gan

Rhyming Round Malaysia by Kathleen Chia and Linda Gan

Rhyming Round Singapore by Kathleen Chia and Linda Gan

Swimmy by Leo Leonni

The Gingerbread Man

The Great Big Enormous Turnip by Alexei Tolstoy

The Three Bears

We're Going on a Bear Hunt by Michael Rosen

Whistle for Willie by Ezra Jack Keats

Who Sank the Boat? by Pamela Allen

Books to Promote Cognitive Development

Brain Games for Preschoolers by Dorothy Einon

Fun for Kids in Singapore by Karen J Renner

Perceptive Play! The A–Z of Discerning Fun for Tots and Parents by Wong Li Lin

Things to Do to Play and Learn by Dorothy Einon

This Little Puffin by Elizabeth M Matterson

Books Dealing with Social and Emotional Issues

The Loss of a Person

Help Me Say Goodbye by Janis L Silverman

Little Bear's Grandad by Nigel Gray

The Goodbye Boat by Mary Joslin

The Death of a Pet

Goodbye Mog by Judith Kerr

Lovely Old Roly by Michael Rosen

Up in Heaven by Emma Chichester

A New Baby in the Family

I'm a Big Brother by Joanna Cole

I'm a Big Sister by Joanna Cole

My New Baby by Annie Kubler

The New Baby at Your House by Joanna Cole

Topsy and Tim: The New Baby by Jean Adamson (The *Topsy and Tim* series of books also deals with many topics that are of concern for a young child like going into hospital, visiting the doctor and dentist, going to school and learning to be safe on the road.)

Waiting for Baby by Annie Kubler

Moving Home and School

Saying Goodbye, Saying Hello... When Your Family is Moving by Michaelene Mundy

Social and Emotional Development

A Kiss Like This by Catherine and Laurence Anholt

Cleversticks by Bernard Ashley

Friend Frog by Alma Flor Ada

Laura's Star by Klaus Baumgart

Max and the Magic Word by Jacqui and Colin Hawkins

New Friends, True Friends, Stuck Like-Glue Friends by Virginia Kroll

Off to School, Baby Duck by Amy Hess

Oh My Baby, Little One by Kathi Appelt

The Ugly Duckling by Hans Christian Andersen

When Sophie Gets Angry—Really, Really Angry by Molly Bang

Food and Nutrition Advice and Recipes

Feed Your Child Right: The First Complete Nutrition Guide for Asian Parents by Lynn Alexander and Yeong Boon Yee

First Foods: Expert Advice and Easy Recipes by Dietitians for Parents of 6–24-Month Olds by Anna Jacob, Pauline Chan, Samantha Thiessen, Janie Chua and Wong Yuefen

Smart Foods for Tweens by Anna Jacob and Ng Hooi Lin

WEBSITES

Helping Your Child to Read

www.ag.ndsu.edu
(Search for "Ages and Stages of Young Readers")

www.booktrustchildrensbooks.org.uk
(Includes children's booklists)

www.kidbibs.com
(Search for "Grow a Reader Booklist")

www.literacytrust.org.uk

www.nwt.literacy.ca
(See "Supporting Children's Literacy Development at Different Ages and Stages")

Interactive Software and Resources

http://ictearlyyears.e2bn.org

General Parenting Articles

www.smartmums.com.sg

www.TheAsianParent.com

TOY SHOPS AND BOOKSTORES

Bookaburra, The Forum

Select Books, Tanglin Shopping Centre

Tango Mango, Tanglin Mall

www.elc.com

www.elc.sg

www.mygrowingtoys.com

www.nurturecraft.com.sg

www.rent-that-toy.com

www.toyrentalworld.com

www.toys4rent.sg

MOTHER AND BABY SUPPLY STORES

Baby's Hyperstore
69 Kaki Bukit Avenue 1, Shun Li Industrial Park
Tel: (65) 6844 1123

Mums & Babes Pte Ltd
www.mumsandbabes.com.sg

About the Contributors

Assoc Prof Daniel Goh, Consultant

Assoc Prof Daniel Goh trained in paediatrics in Singapore and underwent subspecialty training in paediatric pulmonology and sleep at the Johns Hopkins Children's Centre, USA. He currently heads the Paediatric Pulmonary, Sleep and Critical Care Services at the National University Hospital, Singapore, and is the Founding Chairman of the Children's Asthma and Allergy Network, better known as the I CAN! programme (a comprehensive programme for the management of asthma and allergies in children). He is also the current President of the Singapore Paediatric Society and the Vice-President of the College of Paediatrics and Child Health, Singapore. Assoc Prof Goh sits on multiple committees and advisory boards at institutional and national levels, including the National Healthcare Group Institutional Review Board (IRB), Ministry of Health (Singapore) disease management subcommittee on asthma as well as many other professional workgroups. He is also a reviewer for many regional as well as international peer-reviewed journals. He is a Fellow of the Royal College of Paediatrics and Child Health (UK) and a Fellow of the College of Chest Physicians (USA). His clinical interests include childhood respiratory conditions including childhood asthma and allergies, sleep-related breathing disorders in children as well as paediatric bronchology and fibreoptic bronchoscopy. Assoc Prof Daniel Goh is the father of three lovely boys (one a teenager). He loves children and enjoys spending time with them.

Ms Gloria Chan, Writer

Ms Gloria Chan has over 30 years of journalistic experience. She worked as a newspaper reporter for 9 years, then took a break for 5 years to be a full-time mother before rejoining the same organisation, this time working on a parenting magazine as a feature writer for 7 years, covering mostly health, education and parenting matters. She then joined a public health care cluster to start a health magazine that is still in publication today. A mother of two grown-up sons, Ms Chan has since stopped working full-time to write freelance and have more time for herself. As a freelancer, she writes mostly about health care for magazines and health care organisations. For almost two years, Ms Chan wrote a monthly column called Wiser Parent for a magazine, sharing her parenting experience with readers. For this book, she worked with the various expert writers to develop their contributions.

Dr Peter Chew is a senior consultant obstetrician and gynaecologist, infertility specialist and male infertility specialist. He runs a private practice at Gleneagles Hospital. Dr Chew's subspecialty interest is in reproductive medicine, and he has been actively involved in the teaching and training of postgraduate doctors in the clinical management of subfertility, both locally and regionally. He has published widely in this area in peer-reviewed journals and has also written brochures and books for the Ministry of Community Development, Youth and Sports, and articles for female magazines, the *Straits Times*' medical supplement, *Mind Your Body* and *Lianhe Wanbao*, addressing the public on topics pertaining to sexuality and fertility issues. Dr Chew is also a resource speaker for public seminars, talks and TV forums, and has been interviewed on numerous programmes on MediaCorp TV's Channel 5, Channel 8, Channel U, Suria and Channel News Asia. In 2002, Dr Chew founded a non-profit voluntary welfare organisation (VWO), aLife, with a group of other professionals. He currently serves as aLife's chairman and is also a committee member of the I Love Children charity organisation.

Mrs Kathleen Chia married into a Straits-born Chinese family and subsequently raised two children in Singapore. She is a teacher, teacher educator, writer and early years' consultant and holds a teaching qualification and a Master's degree in Child Development with Early Childhood Education from the University of London. While she has lived most of her life in Singapore, she has also lived and worked in Malaysia and the UK. Mrs Chia is a qualified parenting course leader and has conducted parenting courses in the UK and in Singapore. She has also been involved in setting up and volunteering in toy libraries and helping with reading and phonics programmes. Her interest in furthering the development and interests of children with special needs has led to a long and continuing involvement with the Asian Women's Welfare's school for children with disabilities. She now has grandchildren with whom to share her love of stories and rhymes. Mrs Chia has written and published numerous books and learning materials for young children.

Dr Chng Seo Yi is a co-medical director at the Singapore Baby and Child Clinic (SBCC), Lung, Sleep and Allergy Centre in Gleneagles Hospital, Singapore. Prior to joining SBCC, she held the position of consultant paediatrician with the Pulmonology and Sleep Service of the Department of Paediatrics in the National University Hospital and was also an assistant professor and clinical teacher at the Yong Loo Lin School of Medicine, National University of Singapore, where she was involved in teaching and training medical students, junior paediatricians and family physicians. Dr Chng's interests are in childhood asthma and childhood sleep disorders, and she is presently serving as the honorary secretary of the Singapore Sleep Society. She has also published extensively in the areas of allergy, asthma, respiratory infections and sleep disordered breathing.

Dr Chong Shang Chee graduated from the medical faculty of the National University of Singapore in 1998. She obtained her specialist degrees in paediatrics from the Royal College of Paediatrics and Child Health (UK) and Master of Medicine, Paediatrics (Singapore), in 2002. She completed her advanced specialist training in 2005 and currently heads the Child Development Unit (CDU), Division of Development and Behavioural Paediatrics at the University Children's Medical Institute. In 2009, she did a six-month clinical and research attachment at the learning disabilities clinic of the Children's Hospital Boston, Harvard Medical School. She has particular interests in autism, development and behavioural issues, and learning and developmental difficulties in children. She currently heads various programmes at CDU, including helping to pilot a parent-training programme for young toddlers with autism and the preterm neurodevelopmental follow-up programme. She also runs clinics at the Children's Clinic @ Level 4 and the Child Development Unit @ Jurong Medical Centre. Dr Chong has been awarded the Excellent Service Award (EXSA, Silver) in 2005 and the Best Project Prize in the 2005 NHG Clinical Practice Improvement Programme. She strongly advocates for children and families with special needs. She is the mother of two young children.

Asst Prof Linda Gan is married to a Singaporean Chinese and has been living in Singapore for 30 years, subsequently raising her only son here. She holds a Master's degree in Child Development from the University of London and has been lecturing in the Division of Early Childhood and Special Needs at the National Institute of Education, training pre-, primary and secondary school teachers for the past 29 years. During this time, she has been a consultant to the Ministry of Education (MOE) and the Ministry of Community Development, Youth and Sports (MCYS), developing early childhood curricula and preschool teacher training programmes. She is actively involved in supporting children from dysfunctional families in her role as chairperson of the Child Development Committee at Ang Mo Kio Family Service Centre. She has written and published a wide variety of books and enrichment materials for young children.

Ms Anna Jacob is a nutritionist and dietitian with over 26 years of experience in Singapore. She is currently the Nutrition Science and Communications Manager of Abbott Nutrition International, a division of Abbott Laboratories (Singapore) Private Limited. Ms Jacob is also a Board Member of the Singapore Heart Foundation and a Member of the Asia Research and Development Team of Abbott Nutrition Research and Development Centre, Biopolis, Singapore. Ms Jacob earned a bachelor's degree in Nutrition and Dietetics and master's degree in Food Service Management and Dietetics from the Women's Christian College, Madras, India. She is also a full member of the Singapore Nutrition and Dietetics Association (SNDA), the local professional organisation in which she has held the posts of editor and president. Prior to joining Abbott, she was a founding partner and director of Food and Nutrition Specialists P L, a nutrition consultancy firm set up in Singapore in 1989. During this period, she also served as the Associate Director, Scientific Programs for the International Life Sciences Institute Southeast Asia Region (ILSI SEAR). Ms Jacob is a co-author of *First Foods*, *Smart Foods for Tweens* and *Fit Not Fat*, published by Marshall Cavendish International (Asia) Pte Ltd. She has a grown-up daughter.

Sr Kang Phaik Gaik is the

manager/senior lactation consultant at the Parentcraft Centre at Mount Alvernia Hospital. She has been with Mount Alvernia Hospital since 1980 and started the hospital's Parentcraft/Lactation Unit in 1994, which she continues to helm today. Besides running parentcraft and breastfeeding education programmes at the hospital, Sr Kang also conducts public talks for parents-to-be and trains nurses and medical professionals for the Association for Breastfeeding Advocacy (Singapore), or ABAS. Sr Kang was trained in the College of Nursing & Midwifery at Ninewells Hospital, Dundee, Scotland, and became an International Board Certified Lactation Consultant in 1997 and a Certified Infant Massage Instructor in 2007. She has been a Member of the Breastfeeding Mothers' Support Group, Singapore since 1995; Executive Committee Member of the

ABAS since 2003 and President of the International Association for Infant Massage Chapter Singapore since July 2009. Sr Kang is also a workgroup member for the Ministry of Health, which develops Clinical Practice Guidelines on Management of Breastfeeding for healthy full-term infants and premature infants. These guidelines aim to serve as a guide for doctors and nurses in breastfeeding management.

Dr Jennifer Kiing trained at the

University of Melbourne and became a Fellow of the Royal Australasian College of Physicians in 2001. Her general paediatric training was undertaken in part at the Royal Children's Hospital, Melbourne, the Women's and Children's Hospital, Adelaide, and the National University Hospital (NUH), Singapore. Her special interest in developmental and behavioural paediatrics was fostered during a Fellow year spent in community paediatrics at the Centre for Community Child Health, Royal Children's Hospital, Melbourne. She moved to Singapore in March 2000 and is currently a consultant in the Child Development Unit at NUH. She is part of the team that runs the developmental and behavioural paediatrics programme at the Children's Clinic @ Level 4 in NUH as well as Jurong Medical Centre. Her special interests are developmental and behavioural problems in young children, learning difficulties and sleep disorders. Dr Kiing is the mother of three young girls, two of which are twins.

Dr Yvonne Ng is currently a consultant in the Department of Neonatology at the National University Hospital (NUH) and an assistant professor in the Department of Paediatrics, Yong Loo Lin School of Medicine, NUH, with an active role in teaching medical undergraduates and supervising paediatric trainees. She believes strongly in family-centred care, which emphasises close communication and cooperation between the family and health care team for improved patient outcome, and is the medical advisor of the Early Starters Club, a support group for parents of preterm babies at NUH. She is actively involved in improving patient safety and clinical quality as the department's clinical director and patient safety officer. She is also a Clinical Practice Improvement Programme (CPIP) facilitator with the National Healthcare Group, Singapore. Dr Ng is a strong advocate of breastfeeding and is an International Board Certified Lactation Consultant (IBCLC) and the current vice-president of the Association for Breastfeeding Advocacy (Singapore) or ABAS.

Prof Quak Seng Hock is currently professor of paediatrics, Yong Loo Lin School of Medicine, National University of Singapore, and senior consultant, Department of Paediatrics, University Children's Medical Institute, National University Hospital (NUH). He also heads the division of Gastroenterology and Hepatology and is the senior paediatric hepatologist of the Paediatric Liver Transplant Programme at NUH. He was a founder member of the Royal College of Paediatrics and Child Health (UK) and also the founder President of the College of Paediatrics and Child Health, Singapore. He has been practising as a paediatrician since 1979 and his special interests are in children with abdominal pain, diarrheal diseases and childhood cholestasis. He is actively involved in teaching both undergraduate and postgraduate students.

Dr Pamela Sharpe arrived in Singapore in 1985 with her husband and two young sons and was employed at the Institute of Education, now the National Institute of Education (NIE), part of Nanyang Technological University. She obtained a PhD in Child Development from the University of London Institute of Education in 1987 and taught numerous child development, special education and early childhood courses during her time at NIE. She is a founder member of the committee that set up the Rainbow Centre, a special needs school catering to children with intellectual disabilities. She retired from NIE in 2003 and now lives half a year in Malaysia and half a year in the UK. She continues to write book chapters and journal articles on all aspects of early childhood education and acts as consultant to Ngee Ann Polytechnic's Early Childhood and Early Intervention Programmes, the Institute of Technical Education's Higher Nitec Programme in

Early Childhood Education and the joint NIE/Mendaki Project on Early Intervention of Malay Preschool Teachers in Promoting Children's Mathematics Learning. Now a grandmother of two small boys, Dr Sharpe finds herself revisiting the parenting skills she honed many years ago.

Assoc Prof Lynette Shek is a senior consultant paediatrician at the National University Hospital (NUH), Singapore. She trained in allergy, immunology and rheumatology under Prof Lee Bee Wah at NUH, then went to Mount Sinai School of Medicine, New York, for a fellowship from 2002 to 2003. There, she trained with Prof Hugh Sampson, a world-renowned expert in food allergy, and also spent time training in paediatric rheumatology with Prof T Lehman at the Hospital for Special Surgery, New York. She has published in the fields of food allergy and asthma epidemiology, and her subspecialty interests include allergy, immunology and rheumatology.

Dr Wendy Sinnathamby is a specialist in paediatric medicine and is currently attached to the Raffles Children's Centre at Raffles Hospital where she sees patients with a wide variety of general paediatric problems, performs developmental assessments and gives vaccinations. Dr Sinnathamby underwent her undergraduate medical training at United Medical and Dental Schools of Guy's and St Thomas' Hospitals in the UK and went on to complete her postgraduate training in paediatric medicine in the UK, working mainly in South East London and Kent. After completing her postgraduate training in 2004, she was employed as a consultant in general and ambulatory paediatrics at Medway Maritime Hospital, UK, for just over two years. Dr Sinnathamby relocated to Singapore in early 2007 when she joined the University Children's Medical Institute at the National University Hospital (NUH) as consultant in general and ambulatory paediatrics and adolescent medicine. Having lived and worked both in the UK and in Singapore, Dr Sinnathamby is well versed with problems and issues faced by parents across various cultures. Being a parent of a nine-year-old girl herself, she is able to fully empathise with parents and carers and does her best to provide holistic care and advice for her patients.

Dr Mas Suhaila Isa received her medical training from the Yong Loo Lin School of Medicine at the National University of Singapore (NUS) and her Membership of the Royal College of Paediatrics and Child Health (MRCPCH) from the UK. She is currently undergoing further subspecialty training in paediatric infectious disease. Her other areas of interests include immuno-compromised conditions as well as vaccinology. She is a mother of a two-year-old daughter.

Abbott is a global, broad-based health care company devoted to the discovery, development, manufacturing and marketing of pharmaceuticals and medical products, including nutritionals, devices and diagnostics. The company employs nearly 90,000 people and markets its products in more than 130 countries. Abbott began operations in Singapore in 1970 and today has more than 800 employees in the country. Singapore is the regional headquarters for many of Abbott's divisions, as well as a manufacturing and research and development centre for the company.

Abbott Nutrition International, Singapore has been providing science-based nutritional products to support growth, health and wellness for children and adults in Singapore since 1970. As the market leader in paediatric and adult nutrition sector products, Abbott Nutrition feeds over a third of Singapore's children and meets the nutritional needs of adults.